D0943859

DISEASE
LIFE
and
MAN

Stanford Studies in the
Medical Sciences, IX

Disease, Life, and Man

SELECTED ESSAYS BY RUDOLF VIRCHOW

TRANSLATED AND WITH AN INTRODUCTION BY

LELLAND J. RATHER

Stanford University Press

STANFORD, CALIFORNIA

1958

The Library of Congress has cataloged this book as follows:

Virchow, Rudolf Ludwig Karl, 1821–1902.
    Disease, life, and man, selected essays. Translated and with an introd. by Lelland J. Rather. Stanford, Calif., Stanford University Press, 1958.
    x, 273 p. 23 cm. (Stanford studies in the medical sciences, 9)
    Bibliographical references included in "Notes" (p. 247–264)

    1. Medicine—Addresses, essays, lectures. 2. Pathology—Addresses, essays, lectures. 3. Life (Biology)—Addresses, essays, lectures.
    I. Title.   (Series)

R117.V5   610.4   58–13534

Library of Congress

STANFORD UNIVERSITY PRESS
STANFORD, CALIFORNIA
LONDON: OXFORD UNIVERSITY PRESS

© 1958 BY THE BOARD OF TRUSTEES OF THE
LELAND STANFORD JUNIOR UNIVERSITY
ALL RIGHTS RESERVED

PRINTED IN THE UNITED STATES OF AMERICA

610
V81dEr

TO MY CHILDREN

Patricia, Leland, Noel

90312

Preface

Medicine is as old as human society, and man has always attempted to understand and deal with disease in the same terms in which he attempts to understand himself and his creations. Ideas of the nature of disease share in the development of, and reciprocally influence, the ideas of the nature of life and man characteristic of a culture at any given time. In these essays by Rudolf Virchow we can observe the development, reflected in an idea of disease still dominant, of that peculiarly objectified view of life and man so characteristic of modern Western culture. Virchow's theory of the nature of disease, and his insistence on the necessity of applying the scientific method to the study of life and man, both reflected and contributed to a habit of thought beginning to obtain dominance in his own time. He reduced disease to what he considered its core of actuality, and it became, in his eyes, a physical, chemical, or anatomical disturbance of the fundamental units of life—the cells. His conception of scientific method, with its emphasis on objectivity, experimentation, the need for properly placing scientific questions, and the right use of hypotheses, is very close to that of the present day. While still a very young man he began to expound his views in a journal which he himself shared in founding. Then, for fifty-seven years, he stood at the forefront of European medicine. At the same time he attained eminence in politics, where he was a liberal opponent of Bismarck, and in archeology, social medicine, and anthropology. This book contains his views on the nature of disease, life, and man set forth in both technical articles and articles intended for the educated public, since it was part of his credo that medicine should be a cultural force in the life of a people, a form of *paideia*, as it was among the ancient Greeks.

"Standpoints in Scientific Medicine (1847)" and "Standpoints in Scientific Medicine (1877)" were published is the *Bulletin of the History of Medicine* in 1956, and a part of "Scientific Medicine and Therapeutic Standpoints" appeared in the *Stanford Medical Bulletin* in the same year. I have since revised my translations. None of the other essays have appeared in English, as far as I know, with the exception of the Croonian and Huxley lectures. These were published, under titles differing slightly from those I have used, in the *Proceedings of the Royal Society of London* in 1893 and the *British Medical Journal* in 1898, respectively. In view of divergencies between the German and English versions, I have chosen to retranslate both essays from the German. The part of my introductory essay dealing with Virchow was published in the A.M.A. *Archives of Internal Medicine* in 1957, although I have revised the text since.

In preparing these translations I enjoyed the benefit of many suggestions regarding the precise meaning of Virchow's phraseology and my rendering of it from Dr. Ingeborg Arnold, without whose aid and encouragement the book would hardly have come into being. Finally, I wish to thank the personnel of the Stanford University Press, in particular Mr. Jesse G. Bell, Jr., for painstaking, accurate, and helpful editorial assistance.

L. J. R.

Contents

Harvey, Virchow, Bernard, and the Methodology of Science

L. J. Rather, M.D.

IT HAS FREQUENTLY been asserted that natural science is properly inductive, and should proceed from the particular facts of experience to the determination of general laws describing or comprehending these facts. The laws, theories, and hypotheses of science appear, from this point of view, to be the subjective, man-made, part of science, while the "facts" are independent and objectively valid. This interpretation flourished in the nominalistic climate of the English-speaking countries, although it apparently took root less firmly on the European continent. While in the naïve version it has no standing among theorists of scientific method today, it is still effective in an underground fashion and probably accounts in part for the low level of esteem accorded by medical scientists to the construction of theories in comparison with what is called "getting at the facts." Such an attitude toward scientific endeavor has certain harmful effects. Half-hearted and uncritical theoretical work is favored, since theories are taken seriously only as generators of "facts" and are therefore not likely to be criticized acutely. Furthermore—and this is a more serious drawback—this attitude allows large blocks of concealed theory or hypothesis to go unexamined, since the investigator insensitive to theory is likely to be unaware of his own presuppositions, as well as of those of others. Biological and medical scientists are prone to regard discussions of scientific methodology as mere rationalizations made by speculative amateurs. But it is a matter of historical record that some very prominent investigators have concerned themselves with problems in this field. The aim of the present essay is to discuss the ideas of three such men, William Harvey (1578–1657), Claude Bernard (1813–78), and Rudolf Virchow (1821–1902).

William Harvey and the Problem of Knowledge

William Harvey was a younger contemporary of Francis Bacon. Bacon's "new method" seems to have found little favor with Harvey, however, if we are to judge from his comment that Bacon wrote philosophy like a Lord Chancellor. More to the point is the fact that in the introduction to one of Harvey's treatises, in which the problem "of the manner and order of acquiring knowledge" is considered in some detail, Bacon is not even mentioned, nor is there anything in what is said to suggest that Harvey had taken cognizance of Bacon's philosophy of science. Harvey believed that a departure from the then current method of acquiring knowledge was necessary, but he was no despiser of the ancients. He wrote, in fact, that "everything we possess of note or credit in philosophy has been transmitted to us through the industry of ancient Greece." Like Bacon, Harvey had reached the conclusion that knowledge was being pursued in an erroneous and foolish manner in his own time—"so many inquiring what others have said and omitting to ask whether the things be so or not"—and his new way to knowledge was to question things themselves rather than the books of the philosophers. This new way was also a return to the true path. For the ancient philosophers themselves worked in this way "with unwearied labor and variety of experiments." And Aristotle himself advised us, Harvey points out, to ignore what he has written if it conflicts with subsequent observations.

There is only one road to knowledge, according to Harvey, that on which we proceed from things more known to things less known. Science originates by syllogistic reasoning from universals, which are more known to us, to particulars. Here he follows Plato. This emphasis on the role of universals and the importance of syllogistic reasoning was, however, balanced by a favorable evaluation of the inductive procedure. Quoting the opinion of Aristotle that the "whole" is more obvious to our senses, that the "universal is a certain whole," and that it is necessary to proceed from particulars to universals—the way of induction—as well as from universals to particulars, he writes:

All this agrees with what we have previously said, although at first blush it may seem contradictory; inasmuch as universals are first imbibed from particulars by the senses, and in so far are only known to us as an universal is a certain whole and indistinct thing, and a whole is known to us according to sense. For though in all knowledge we begin from sense, because, as the philosopher quoted has it, sensible particulars are better known to sense, still the sensation itself is an universal thing. For, if you observe rightly, although in the external sense the object perceived is singular, as for example, the colour which we call yellow in the eye, still when this impression comes to be made an abstraction, and to be judged of and understood by the internal sensorium, it is an universal. Whence it happens that several persons abstract several species, and conceive different notions, from viewing the same object at the same time. This is conspicuous among poets and painters, who, although they contemplate one and the same object in the same place at the same movement, and with all other circumstances agreeing, nevertheless regard and describe it variously, and as each has conceived or formed an idea of it in his imagination. In the same way the painter having a certain portrait to delineate, if he draw the outline a thousand times, he will still give it a different face, and each not only differing from the other, but from the original countenance; with such slight variety, however, that looking at them singly, you shall conceive you have still the same portrait set before you, although, when set side by side, you perceive how different they are.[1]

In the above illustration the different delineations, all of which resemble the original face, represent particular instances of an universal. Harvey then proceeds to elaborate Seneca's distinction of the *Eidos* from the *idea*, and to draw an interesting parallel between the work of the artist and the work of the scientist. The artist *imitates* the pattern, prototype, or idea, but he *creates* the Eidos, species, or representation. Harvey continues:

On the same terms, therefore, as art is attained to, is all knowledge and science acquired; for as art is a habit with reference to things to be done, so is science a habit in respect of things to be known: as that proceeds from the imitation of types or forms, so this proceeds from the knowledge of natural things. Each has its origin in sense and ex-

---

[1] Notes will be found on pp. 247–63.

perience, and it is impossible that there can rightly be either art or science without visible instance or example. In both, that which we perceive in sensible objects differs from the image itself which we retain in our imagination or memory. That is the type, idea, forma informans; this is the imitation, the Eidos, the abstract species. That is a thing natural, a real entity; this a representation or similitude, and a thing of the reason. That is occupied within the individual thing, and itself is single and particular; this a certain universal and common thing. That in the artist and man of science is a sensible thing, clear, more perfect; this a matter of reason and more obscure: for things perceived by sense are more assured and manifest than matters inferred by reason, inasmuch as the latter proceed from and are illustrated by the former. Finally, sensible things are of themselves and antecedent; things of the intellect, however, are consequent, and arise from the former, and indeed, we can in no way attain to them without the help of the others. And hence it is, that without the due admonition of the senses, without frequent observation and reiterated experiment, our mind goes astray after phantoms and appearances.[2]

Harvey's procedure is Aristotelian in its emphasis on the priority of the syllogistic method and the necessity for working back to first principles. He makes no hypotheses in terms of invisible entities, whose effects alone are visible, as the modern scientist often does, nor does he use the "hypothetical method" of Plato, in which a postulate or thesis is put forward and a system evolved by deductive reasoning.[3] The order by which any art or science is acquired is as follows:

The thing perceived by sense remains; from the permanence of the thing perceived results memory; from multiplied memory, experience; from experience, universal reasons, definitions, and maxims or common axioms, the most certain principles of knowledge; for example, the same thing under like conditions cannot be and not be; every affirmation or negation is either true or false; and so on.[4]

In his studies on the circulation of the blood and generation in animals Harvey does not seem to seek for explanations so much as for clear-cut, logically sound descriptions of what actually happens. Both works, the latter in particular, are masterpieces of natural-scientific description, and in reading them it is easy to overlook the explanatory hypotheses inserted among the generalizations from observation. The chief hypothesis in Harvey's *De Motu Cordis* is that the heart is a propelling organ which drives the blood in a double circle through the lungs and the rest of the body. Willis states that the first part of the hypothesis was as much a novelty as the second, and Woodger points out that this was probably responsible for the great resistance encountered by Harvey's ideas.[5] For, if the pumping action of the heart is accepted, Harvey's arguments for the occurrence of a circular movement of the blood become almost irresistible. On the other hand, if the heart is regarded as a kind of retort or pressure cooker, various other hypotheses may be brought forward to explain his demonstrations.[6] It is worth noting that Harvey's hypothesis was of a kind that could be directly verified. By directly, I mean that the hypothesis itself—not only its consequences—was verifiable in its own terms. Ordinarily by "verification" we mean only that the predicted consequences of our hypothetical assertions can be shown to occur. The hypothetical assertion is the antecedent of the scientific argument, and the experimental or observational result is the consequent. The argument has the form of the hypothetical syllogism "If A, then B." But to assert that A is true simply because B is true is to commit the fallacy of the consequent. Because of the inconclusive character of verification the "falsifiability" criterion was brought forward as a means for coping with the difficulty, but it is at best of negative value. The further attempt to change the conditional argument into a biconditional of the form "If, and only if, A, then B" is not scientifically feasible. But to claim, as Woodger does,[7] that Harvey's hypothesis is still a hypothesis today—since "once a hypothesis, always a hypothesis"—does not take into account the modern techniques of observation. It is now possible to insert catheters directly into the chambers of the heart and measure the systolic and diastolic pressures; one can also see the movement of the blood in the great arteries, using the fluoroscope and injecting radio-opaque dyes into the circulation. It is even possible to bypass the heart entirely and put a mechanical pump in its place.[8]

The existence of the capillary circulation, and the absence of "pores" in the interventricular septum, can also be directly demonstrated today, whereas in Harvey's time this was not possible. In the epistemological discussion which prefaces his *De Generatione* Harvey is concerned with the traditional problem of the relation between universals and particulars. The problem of justifying the use of hypotheses does not arise, and is nowhere taken up in his writings. As we have seen, however, he does make hypotheses. Two of these, the circulation of the blood and the source of its movement in the muscular contraction of the heart, have been directly verified; one other, the explanation of diastole in terms of expansion of the blood due to its innate heat (in a manner analogous to fermentation), has been discarded. And the problem of the right relation between universals and particulars still remains with us, in spite of the attempts made by linguistic analysts and positivists to reduce it to a pseudo or nonsense question.

Claude Bernard and Experimental Medicine

Claude Bernard did not publish on the topic of methodology until he was a well-established scientific investigator. The *Introduction to the Study of Experimental Medicine*, his first treatment of the subject, appeared in 1865, when Bernard was fifty-three years of age. The book was well received at the time of its publication, and grew steadily in repute until several decades later Bergson compared it favorably with Descartes' "Discourse on Method."[9] Bernard's avowed purpose in writing the book was to further the cause of scientific medicine through an investigation of the principles of experimental research. He believed that an experimenter must be a theorist as well as a practitioner, possessing a clear understanding of the principles which guide his reasoning in the study of natural phenomena. In his emphasis on the necessity of a philosophical approach to the problems of science, as well as in his neovitalistic outlook, Bernard was one step removed from the positivistic bias of most of his contemporaries in the nineteenth-century world of science.[10]

Bernard begins with a discussion of the interrelationships of observation, experience, and experiment. Both observers and experimenters bring forward new facts for rational consideration, and the method of experimental reasoning is the same in both the "observational" and "experimental" sciences. Observation and experiment stand at the two poles of experimental reasoning, as it were, and the degree of difference is determined by the extent to which the scientific worker alters and controls the factors influencing the natural phenomena which he seeks to understand. The experimental method used in science is no more than a refinement of experience, the one source of human knowledge. "Experience," Bernard writes, quoting Goethe, "disciplines us every day." Scientists correct their scientific ideas on the basis of experience, bringing them more in harmony with the facts and thus nearer to the truth. The knowledge we gain from everyday experience is necessarily accompanied by vague experimental reasoning, carried on quite unawares, in consequence of which judgments are made about facts. But this "marche obscure et spontanée de l'esprit" can be developed into a method which proceeds rapidly and consciously toward a definite goal.

There are two separable operations in the experimental method: the planning of the experiment itself and the noting of the results. The first operation requires preconceived ideas; the second must avoid them at all costs. The blind naturalist François Huber was able to devise admirable experiments on bees, which were afterwards carried out and described for him by a serving man who had no scientific ideas whatsoever. This is a paradigm for the right method of procedure, since:

It is impossible to devise an experiment without a preconceived idea; devising an experiment, we said, is putting a question; we never conceive a question without an idea which invites an answer. I consider it, therefore, an absolute principle that experiments must always be devised in view of a preconceived idea, no matter if the idea be not very clear nor very well defined. As for noting the results of the experiment, which is itself only an induced observation, I posit it similarly as a principle that we must here, as always, observe without a preconceived idea.[11]

The condemnation of hypotheses and *a priori* ideas rests, according to Bernard, on a failure to distinguish between the observational procedure, whether in the clinic or in the laboratory, and the questions in the mind of the observer or experimenter which lead him to turn his attention and activities in a definite direction. Men who merely gather observations further the cause of science only in so far as their observations are afterward introduced into experimental reasoning, and men who experiment cannot solve problems unless their work is inspired by a fortunate hypothesis; on the other hand, hypotheses based on observations fathered by others are useful only in so far as they are subjected to the experimental test. Unverified and unverifiable hypotheses engender systems and lead back to scholasticism. The metaphysician and the experimental reasoner both work with *a priori* ideas, but the former posits his idea as an absolute and proceeds to deduce its consequences, while the latter "states an idea as a question, as an interpretative, more or less probable anticipation of nature, from which he logically deduces consequences which, moment by moment, he confronts with reality by means of experiment."[12]

Bacon, wrote Bernard, was not a man of science and he did not understand the experimental method, as his own fruitless attempts sufficiently demonstrate. Bacon advises the investigator to fly from theories and hypotheses, and entirely fails to see that these are as necessary as the scaffolding of a house. The Baconian emphasis on induction is understandable as a reaction against the systematic deductive procedure of the scholastics, but the distinction between induction and deduction is not useful in the elucidation of the experimental method. If induction is defined as the process of moving from the particular to the general, and deduction as the reverse process of moving from the general to the particular:

. . . I shall content myself with saying that it seems to me very difficult in practice to justify this distinction and clearly to separate induction from deduction. If the experimenter's mind usually proceeds by starting from particular observations and going back to principles, to laws, or to general propositions, it also necessarily proceeds from the same general propositions or laws and reaches particular facts which it deduces logically from these principles. . . . It would be incorrect to say that deduction pertains only to mathematics and induction to the other sciences exclusively.[13]

Both forms of reasoning are used in all possible sciences, because in all of the sciences there are things that we do not know and other things that we know or think we know. An investigator might start either from a chance observation that he sought to explain, or from a hypothesis that he wanted to test. On observing the clear and acid urine of rabbits brought from the market to his laboratory, Bernard drew the conclusion that the animals must somehow be in the nutritional condition of carnivora (i.e. subsisting on their own protein), since carnivora, too, void clear and acid urine. He proceeded to test his hypothesis by feeding grass to the rabbits, whereupon their urine became cloudy and alkaline. He then fed them boiled beef, and their urine again became acid and clear. He described his reasoning as follows:

The inductive reasoning which I implicitly went through was the following syllogism: the urine of carnivora is acid; now the rabbits before me have acid urine, therefore they are carnivora, i.e. fasting. This remained to be established by experiment.[14]

As a matter of fact, the acidity of rabbit urine can be varied independently of the protein intake by varying the mineral content of the diet.

At this point an ambiguity in the meaning of the term induction becomes apparent. If induction is no more than the passing from the particular to the general, as Bernard states, is it legitimate for him to describe his own procedure as inductive, without making it clear that something new has been introduced? The generalization of his observation would have been, simply, that all fasting rabbits voided clear and acid urine. What he offers in addition to a generalization is a hypothetical explanation based on an analogy drawn between carnivorous and herbivorous animals. To reach the level of hypothesis and theory it is necessary to pass at least one step beyond observation generalizations.[15] From the standpoint of linguistic analysis, a standpoint which is unobjectionable if its limitations are understood, this involves the construction of statements of successively higher order. The edifice of a theoretically developed science may be regarded as a pyramid, resting on a foundation of primary experience, consisting of statements of successively higher order of abstraction.[16]

The "something new" referred to in the previous paragraph is based on experience, but on experience which ought to be considered from a broader point of view than that of ordinary empiricism. It involves the creative ability to discern patterns of order and similarity in realms where only confusion and bewilderment are experienced by others. This is, in fact, the original meaning of the Greek word "theory," for it signified a "seeing" in the sense of insight—an act of intellectual vision leading to the discernment of the One in the Many, or, as we would say today, to the recognition of invariant relations in the flux of events. The creation involved is not the spinning of arbitrary fantasies, as all theory appears to be from the viewpoint of extreme nominalism, nor is it simply the proper generalization of particular facts; rather it is that kind of creation which Harvey tried to describe when he wrote that the scientist, as well as the artist, imitates the pattern, but creates the *Eidos*.

Rudolf Virchow and Scientific Medicine

It is no longer necessary today to write that scientific medicine is also the best foundation for medical practice. It is sufficient to point out how completely even the external character of medical practice has changed in the last thirty years. Scientific methods have been everywhere introduced into practice. The diagnosis and prognosis of the physician are based on the experience of the pathological anatomist and the physiologist. Therapeutic doctrine has become biological and thereby experimental science.

—RUDOLF VIRCHOW, 1877

In the arresting image which closes his great book, Marcel Proust envisions the aged Duc de Guermantes as a being perched on ceaselessly growing living stilts, a giant plunged in the years and epochs of the past. So must Virchow have appeared to his friends and associates at the beginning of the twentieth century, two years before his death. As early as 1847 he had founded the

Archiv für pathologische Anatomie und Physiologie und für klinische Medizin. His book *Cellularpathologie,* published in 1858, was without doubt the most influential work on disease to appear in the nineteenth century. Fifty years after having become a full professor of pathological anatomy at Würzburg he was still tirelessly active in medicine; in 1898 he delivered, in English, the second Huxley lecture before a distinguished audience of scientists and notables in London.

Virchow became a person to reckon with in German medical circles at the age of twenty-three when, in a talk given before some of Germany's most prominent civilian and military physicians in Berlin, he successfully attacked the accepted doctrines concerning phlebitis. Shortly thereafter he began a series of lectures on pathological anatomy. These were well received and his name remained in the public eye. In a letter written to his father at this time he offered the following "curious example" to prove this point: At a ball he was dancing with a young woman to whom he had just been introduced. To his surprise she asked him first to repeat, and then to spell, his name, remarking finally that it must be his father who was giving the lectures on pathological anatomy. The young woman simply could not believe that her beardless young dancing partner was the famous Dr. Virchow![17] Fifty-seven years after thus stirring up the medical circles of Berlin, and after distinguishing himself in anthropology, politics, and social medicine as well as in pathology, Virchow died, his physical and mental powers still largely unimpaired.

No one who reads Virchow's scientific and philosophical papers can fail to be impressed by the breadth and power of his mind. But those who know Virchow as a scientist and philosopher—let alone those who know him merely as a pathologist—are acquainted with only one aspect of his activity. He was an archeologist who had excavated with Schliemann at the site of Troy, the author of a book on Trojan graves, who did his own archeological field work in the Caucasus at the age of seventy-three, an anthropologist and ethnologist who edited the *Zeitschrift für Ethnologie* and whose survey of seven million German school children in 1876 should have buried forever the myth of the blond, blue-eyed German race, a linguist who knew English, French, Italian, and Dutch, and worked with Latin, Greek, Hebrew, and Arabic. He was a socially-minded man who said that science should speak the language of the common people and who derided nationalism in science; he was active in politics from his youthful days on the barricades in 1848 to his struggle with Bismarck, as leader of the progressive party in the Prussian diet.

Virchow was a Faustian figure whose aim was "no less than a universal knowledge of nature from Godhead to stone"—as he wrote in a letter to his father at the age of twenty-one. His abilities were even then obvious to his contemporaries. The German medical historian Paul Diepgen quotes a letter written by Leubuscher to Meckel stating that the twenty-four-year-old Virchow had "an undeniable degree of intellectual power and authority, and an astounding ability to keep in mind and integrate all sorts of apparently unrelated observations."[18] The fact is that for Virchow the observations were not at all unrelated. He was the kind of man who sees things in terms of their relationships. Yet he was at the same time probably the most careful and critical medical investigator of his day.

The problem of the proper method of science was one of the first with which he dealt. In Germany in the late eighteenth and early nineteenth centuries, the influence of a strongly idealistic philosophy had led many speculative biologists and medical men to believe that by sheer abstract thought it would be possible to solve the major biological problems. To Virchow, the fatal error of this, the natural-philosophical, school in medicine, lay in an unchecked propensity to erect hypotheses on the basis of the flimsiest kind of evidence and to draw far-reaching analogies in an uncritical fashion. Virchow wanted to relegate hypotheses to a "housebroken" state, he wrote, but he was far from wishing to dispense with them entirely or to ban the use of analogy. He simply wanted critical control exercised in the light of a detailed examination of the facts. With a remarkably clear idea of scientific method, avoiding both the halting gait of narrowly conceived Baconian induction and the erratic flights of the less critical nature-philosophers, he stated that hypotheses and analogies should be firmly based on phenomena of general occurrence. In this case they could function as entering wedges for further investigation. About two decades later, Claude Bernard was to write that hypotheses were indispensable precisely because they led science beyond the facts and thus permitted it to progress. Virchow, long before, had said that a hypothesis should be a scientific question, posed with the aid of induction and analogy, based on known scientific laws. The answer was to be derived from the experiment implied in a properly placed question. Experimentation was the court of last resort.

The inflation of *aperçus*—brilliant or otherwise—into exclusive medical systems claiming to explain all and everything and threatening recalcitrant matters of fact with excommunication is still with us today, but the systems are implicit rather than fully developed. This is a defect, of course, but we may on the other hand credit ourselves with an enormous amount of precise factual information in medicine and the special sciences which contribute to it. Virchow thought that the pressing need of his time was the collection of exactly this kind of data, to be achieved by a careful critical investigation of specific matters of fact— *Detail Untersuchungen*, he called it—and by the suppression of irresponsible theorizing. When one considers the number of conflicting schools in medicine at the time, this reaction is understandable. Walter Pagel, in an informative essay on the speculative basis of modern pathology, quotes the following listing from a slightly older contemporary of Virchow's and a member of the natural-historical school, Ferdinand Jahn:

Metaphysicians, Idealists, Iatromechanics, Iatrochemists, Experimental Physiologists, Natural Philosophers, Mystics, Magnetizers, Exorcisers, Galenists, Modern Paracelsian Homunculi, Stahlianists, Humoral Pathologists, Gastricists, Infarct-Men, Broussaisists, Contrastimulists, Natural Historians, Physiatricists, Ideal-Pathologists, German Christian Theosophists, Schoenleinian Epigones, Pseudo-Schoenleinians, Homeobiotics, Homeopathists, Isopathists, Homeopathic Allopathists, Psorists and Scorists, Hydropathists, Electricity-

Men, Physiologists after Hamberger, Heinrothians, Sachsians, Kieserians, Hegelians, Morisonians, Phrenologists, Iatrostatisticians.[19]

In this listing we recognize many friends still among us. Some lead a twilight existence on the fringes of orthodox medicine. One—the iatrostatistician—has swelled in importance.

Systems, according to Virchow, were to be avoided until a sufficient quantity of empirical data could be accumulated. This point of view is now widely accepted and is certainly valid within limits. Two pertinent comments concerning it may be made, however: first, the point at which a sufficient quantity of empirical data will be available for the purpose of systematization is apt to recede indefinitely, since it soon becomes easier to accumulate facts than to reduce them to order; second, it may be argued that empirical data are never gathered in the absence of a system. Some set of presuppositions about the nature of the world, of man, and of disease will determine the character of the facts to be accumulated. The system may be implied in the procedure of investigation, rather than explicitly proclaimed as a program. The point at which a sufficient quantity of empirical data seems to be available keeps receding because the data always contain a theoretical element. Consequently, when the concealed systematic or theoretical elements change, there is a need for reinterpretation of the data in answer to new questions that arise, as well as a need for additional data bearing on these questions.

Virchow himself developed a system of cellular pathology, basing it, within its limits, quite firmly on careful observation. This system seemed for a while to answer most of the important questions in medicine, or to give promise of eventually answering them. Then, rather suddenly, in connection with a great shift in scientific opinion involving a general devaluation of morphology, the system began to appear worthless to many investigators. The shift should have had less effect than it did, since Virchow's cellular pathology was not simply pathological anatomy, as is so often supposed. In fact, he violently rejected Rokitansky's claim that diseases were at all times open to morphological investigation. Nevertheless, largely owing to technical advances in microscopy

and the staining of cells and tissues, which made the application of the morphological method extraordinarily fruitful in the
study of disease, cellular pathology was somewhat one-sidedly
developed, and in our day is usually confused with pathological
anatomy. But it is neither pathological anatomy, a science which
can be pursued in the absence of any knowledge of cells, nor
pathological histology, nor organ pathology. It is a principle
which has transformed all of these, and in addition a theory of
the nature of disease. Virchow was himself very well aware of the
limitations inherent in a purely anatomical approach. For how,
he wrote in 1849, can one in this way "with certainty decide which
of two coexistent phenomena is the cause and which the effect,
whether one of them is the cause at all instead of both being effects
of a third cause, or even whether both are effects of two entirely
unrelated causes?" The difficulties involved in attempting to
infer temporal and causal relationships from objects known only
in their spatial relationships could hardly be more succinctly
expressed.

The position of Virchow in the history of medical thought is
most frequently misjudged by those who class him with the proponents of what might be called intransigent anatomicism, i.e. the
view that anatomical changes must be at the root of all diseases.
Even in Germany, August Bier, writing in 1937, found it necessary to protest against this misunderstanding and to call attention
to the fact that Virchow regarded cellular pathology as a biological, not a purely anatomical, theory of disease.[20] In 1938,
during a period in which Virchow stood under a cloud because
his ideas of race offended Nazi sensibilities, Ludwig Aschoff once
more protested against such misrepresentations.[21] The statement
that Virchow's cellular pathology is a biological theory of disease
simply means that it treats of disease as a disturbance of the fundamental living unit, the cell. This does not mean that the techniques of physics and chemistry cannot be used in the study of the
cell. On the contrary, their use is called for. But even if living
things were to be explained in terms of the mechanical results of
molecular forces, wrote Virchow, it would still be necessary to
designate with some special name the form in which these forces

are embodied. Our experience, according to Virchow, teaches us that life can manifest itself only in a concrete form, bound to certain substantial loci. These loci are the cells. The cell is at once the fundamental unit of life and the fundamental unit of disease.

An important feature of cellular pathology is the ultimacy of localization. Strictly speaking, Virchow wrote, there are no generalized diseases. All diseases can be localized, since they are bound to cells. Aschoff has argued that Virchow wanted to localize lesions, rather than diseases, basing his contention on a few lines written in 1854: ". . . it is certainly consequent to localize diseases (not disease), and to assign them specific anatomical seats."[22] A distinction, not too plain, is made here between *Krankheiten* and *die Krankheit*. If a distinction had been made between diseases understood as clinical entities and diseases as characterized by cellular lesions, a difficulty that has plagued medical theorists would never have arisen. Perhaps Virchow merely meant that the subjective aspect of disease could not be localized. In any case, he stated quite clearly in the same paper that localization of disease processes does not imply that anatomical or histological changes are necessarily present. It was for this reason, among others, that he opposed the great pathological anatomist Carl Rokitansky:

The basic error of this [Rokitansky's] point of view rests, in our opinion, on the confusion of the anatomical with the material. We are, as well, in no position to conceive of any kind of living process in the human being, regardless of how functional it may seem, without a material change—however, must it therefore be anatomical? . . . Every anatomical change is a material one as well, but is every material change, therefore, also anatomical? Can it not be molecular? Can a deep-reaching molecular alteration of the inner composition of matter not take place with the preservation of its inner form and outer appearance? These finer molecular changes of matter are objects of physiology rather than anatomy; they are functional—dynamic, if one wishes to use this forbidden expression. The stimulated, functioning nerve is anatomically no different from the latently active "resting" nerve; the structure of necrotic bone may completely correspond to that of living bone. One can have the greatest respect for anatomical, morphological, and histological studies, and one can regard them as the unavoidably necessary foundation for all further investigation—but must one proclaim them, therefore, the only ones to be pursued, the ones of exclusive significance? Many important phenomena in the body are of a purely functional kind, and when one attempts to explain these also with a mechanistic hypothesis, in terms of fine-molecular changes, it should never be forgotten that the methods for their observation and pursuit can never be anatomical.[23]

Virchow's conception of disease, then, rests on four chief hypotheses: (1) all diseases are reducible to active or passive disturbances of living cells; (2) all cells arise from parent cells; (3) the functional capacities of cells depend on intracellular physical and chemical processes and may to some extent be inferred from morphological changes; (4) all pathological formations are degenerations, transformations, or repetitions of normal structures. The second of these, often regarded as a fact of observation today, represents Virchow's specific contribution to cell theory. He tells us, in his second essay on standpoints in scientific medicine, that he first entertained it as a "heretical thought" and that it was five years before he began to "break the spell of the cell theory" as then conceived. All four are still hypotheses today.[24]

Virchow and the Ontological Conception of Disease

In his two papers "Standpoints in Scientific Medicine"[25] and "Scientific Methods and Therapeutic Standpoints,"[26] published in 1847 and 1849, respectively, Virchow rejects the ontological conception of disease in favor of the physiological conception. Yet in his paper "One Hundred Years of General Pathology," written forty-five years later, he states that cellular pathology is

. . . expressly ontological. That is its merit, not its deficiency. There actually is an *ens morbi*, just as there is an *ens vitae*; in both instances a cell or cell-complex has the claim to be thus designated. The *ens morbi* is at the same time a parasite in the sense of the natural-historical school, not in the sense of the bacteriologists.[27]

What happened in the interim? The answer to this question will disclose the nature of Virchow's achievement.

The distinction between the ontological and the physiological conception of disease can be made clear in a few words. The essence of the ontological conception is the idea that diseases are substantial things (*entia, onta*), that they have real existence as such. The essence of the physiological conception is that diseases have no existence as such but are merely reflections of deranged function. Where the ontologist sees discrete entities, each with its own peculiar law of development, the physiologist sees quantitative deviations from the normal course of bodily function. Now a great many variations on these two themes are possible. The one that offended Virchow in his younger days was the parasitic theory of disease, particularly as developed by the school of natural historians. In this conception not the etiological agent but the disease process itself was regarded as a parasitic lower life form. A therapeutic corollary was sometimes included. Should there not be a therapeutic entity corresponding to each disease entity? With regard to this, Virchow wrote:

. . . as soon as one is convinced that there are no disease entities one must realize also that no therapeutic entities can be set up in opposition to them. . . . If disease is only the orderly manifestation of definite phenomena of life (normal in themselves) under unusual conditions, with deviations which are simply quantitative, then all therapy must be essentially directed against the altered conditions. . . .[28]

In this period Virchow seemed to be wholly caught up in the great swing toward the physiological conception of disease which was taking place in Germany and France. In his inaugural address at the Collége de France in 1847, Claude Bernard stated that his task would be to develop the physiological basis on which scientific medicine would rest. In the same year, Virchow wrote:

. . . the final decision in these matters belongs to a science which at the present time consists only in rudiments, and which appears destined to replace general pathology; I refer to pathological physiology . . . a pathological physiology which will be the stronghold of scientific medicine, where pathological anatomy and the clinic are only the outworks.[29]

In reality, however, he had in mind a question resting upon an ontological presupposition. The question was simply this: Where is the concrete disease? Where is its seat?[30] The humoral pathologists had placed it in the fluid parts, the solidary pathologists in the solid parts, of the body. Neither answer satisfied Virchow. Both contained incomplete truths and did not suffice for the unitary standpoint that he sought for. He was able to reconcile the conflict between the ontological and physiological conceptions of disease by conceiving of disease as life under abnormal conditions on the one hand and by finding the seat of life in the cell on the other. The concrete representation of disease—without which it remained, he wrote, a shadow picture, a formless thing—was then the deranged cell. Once Virchow had become convinced that cells arose only from preexistent cells, rather than from a formless "blastema" as both Schleiden and Schwann had supposed, the old conflict between solidary and humoral views of life and disease became meaningless. The cell had both solid and fluid parts. Life, though a "movement," was bound to a concrete thing, the living cell.

Another form of the ontological view had been cultivated by the natural-historical school. This had to a large extent originated with Sydenham, in the seventeenth century. According to Sydenham, diseases were definite entities, with their own laws of growth, development, and decline, rather than simply random configurations of pathophysiological events. We had as much reason, he wrote,[31] to consider diseases as discrete species as we had plants. The plant springs from the earth, blooms, and dies. The disease does all this with equal regularity. The only puzzling feature for Sydenham was the apparent lack of "substance" in diseases, since he believed them to be dependent on humoral dyscrasias. We can almost hear Sydenham asking the same question as Virchow asked two hundred years later: Where is the concrete disease?

Sydenham's entity was a "clinical entity," and Virchow's was to become a "pathological entity" which in the minds of many was to give "substance" to the clinical entity—so much so that without a visible lesion in the tissues a later generation of physicians found it difficult to believe that a patient was really ill.

Variations in the ontological view depend on the kind of being accorded to the entities in question, and the whole problem is a subspecies of the problem of universals versus particulars. In a crudely realistic approach (i.e. realistic in the Platonic sense) there is the danger of hypostatization of concepts—the ascription of being to things that have no being which Virchow objected to in 1849[32]—while in thoroughgoing nominalism there is the risk that diseases will be regarded as no more than convenient fictions. Unless an element of order is introduced into the welter of phenomena observable at the sickbed it would be impossible for the clinician to foresee the future course of the patient under his care and thus to govern his treatment. Although to the layman one ill person seems very much like another, to the eye of the clinician there are definite patterns to be descried. Moreover, the clinician has always been reluctant to believe that he himself has introduced the elements of order into the phenomena; he prefers to think that he has only discerned what was already there. Just as the microscopist sees a meaningful pattern of order in his bits of stained tissue, so the clinician sees universal patterns in what seems to the layman a "buzzing blooming confusion," to borrow a phrase of William James.

Linking his work with that of Morgagni in the previous century, Virchow wrote[33] that he had carried to its theoretical conclusion the investigation initiated by his predecessor in the *De Sedibus et Causis Morborum*. In a logically consequent development of Morgagni's "anatomical idea" there had been a progression from the correlation of clinical histories with grossly visible anatomical lesions, through the conception of diseased tissues as developed by Bichat, to the discovery of the ultimate seat of disease in the living cell. A point had been reached where the knife no longer sufficed for the investigation of processes taking place in disease, and the idea of localization had to be enlarged to cover invisible, inferred physico-chemical changes. Clinical entities corresponded to cellular pathological entities, the orderly course of whose events determined the clinical picture. This was Virchow's theoretical triumph.

Virchow and Philosophy

Virchow did not pretend to be an original or profound philosopher, nor did he as a rule pursue his ideas to the bases on which they ultimately rested. Yet it is remarkable to see how explicitly he formulated his views at the outset of his career. The transcendental element in French and German thought and the retreat from Lockean sensualism, which have made the intellectual atmosphere of the European continent so different from that of the Anglo-American countries, apparently had little influence on him. Virchow, it seems, would have been quite at home among the English empiricists. It is easier to imagine him conversing with Mill than with Kant. In *Die Einheitsbestrebungen in der wissenschaftlichen Medicin*, he states that all human understanding is based on an awareness of the relations of the person to what lies beyond him, relations that become known as a result of changes excited in the central nervous system by the sense organs. His "neurological" reduction of culture would have satisfied Hobbes, and is far more radical than Marx's reduction of culture to a dialectical interplay of the forces of production:

The complexity of the relationships of the sense organs to the external world, therefore, determines the extent of intellectual activity and the scope of culture. . . . Culture, however, consists not only in the scope of sensual awareness, but essentially in the energy of the interrelated excitations of the central apparatus, in the communication of excitations from the sensual receptors to numerous groups of ganglion cells.[34]

Science, according to Virchow, commences with the history of material bodies and then enquires into the mechanisms of their origin and development, into temporal and causal relationships, being more concerned with the processes in which they are involved than with the bodies themselves.[35] Whatever is beyond these material bodies and their properties is transcendent, and the scientist regards preoccupation with this sphere as an aberration of the human spirit. Virchow thus appears to be a materialist at first sight. Eleven years later, however, in a lecture before the Deutsche Versammlung Naturforscher und Ärzte devoted to the mechanistic conception of life,[36] he specifically rejects materialism as a system on the ground that it goes beyond our experience and lays the narrow measure of its knowledge on every phenomenon. But this is as far as he will go. There may be something beyond experience, he says, but whatever its nature it is no part of the business of science to be concerned with it. The core of Virchow's philosophy of science lies in his insistence on the rule of causality, necessity, and law in all realms of nature, including the organic world and the human spirit, and his rejection of anything occult or mysterious.

Actually, his views on the nature of life did undergo a perceptible change after he began to concentrate his attention on the living cell, so much so that some of his opponents were led to accuse him of vitalism. What happened was that he discarded the overhasty reduction (made by crude mechanistic materialists of his time) of living processes to simple mechanical movements. In reply to Spiess, a prominent "neural" pathologist whom he respected and whose objections he published in his own *Archiv*, he wrote:

It arouses the concern of Herr Spiess that I have permitted myself the expression "life-force," which I formerly avoided. I have never assumed "special vital forces" as Herr Spiess claims. I do not deny that this has its risks, though not so much on my account as on that of others who think of something quite different from my conception in connection with this word. In the end, however, a term is needed, and it would be impossible to find one that could not be misunderstood or misinterpreted. Nowhere have I even hinted that life-force is primary, or specifically different from the other natural forces; on the contrary, I have repeatedly and emphatically stated the likelihood of its mechanical origin. But it is high time that we give up the scientific prudery of regarding living processes as nothing more than the mechanical resultant of molecular forces inherent in the constitutive particles.[37]

Forty years later he wrote of cellular pathology:

Nothing prevents anyone from calling such an attitude vitalism. It should not, of course, be forgotten that no special life-force can be discovered, and that vitalism in this sense does not of necessity signify either a spiritual or a dynamic system. But it is likewise necessary to understand that life is different from processes in the rest of the world, and cannot be simply reduced to physical or chemical forces.[38]

Like many scientists of his day, Virchow believed that European civilization had progressed from a philosophical to a scientific era. He had never recovered from his reaction against the nature-philosophers of his youth and was apt to consider philosophy as armchair speculation. In 1893 he said that more and more people were beginning to understand that science could only make progress with the aid of museums, laboratories, and institutes. Experiment was the most important means of forcing nature to divulge the character, causes, and sequences of natural processes. No valid conclusions concerning actual natural processes, he said, had come from the study rooms of the philosophers. Virchow must have known that his own idea of the nature of disease had forced a complete revision of medical thought, and it is a little saddening to see him trapped into this vulgar philistinism of expression. The ideas of Virchow himself had come from the study rooms of philosophers. He had given them flesh—a worthy task, but not the whole of it.

But there was another, more understandable, facet to his attitude toward loose "philosophizing" of a certain kind. Animal magnetism, spiritualism, hypnotism, racial mystique, and all manner of unhealthy trends seemed to him to be bound up with an antirational speculative view turning in the direction of a dark and unknown side of the human spirit. In the early part of the nineteenth century the University of Berlin had, for a brief time, two professorships in "animal magnetism." Today (1893), wrote Virchow in noting this, we have to cope with spiritualism and hypnotism. Will science be strong enough to guard against the dangers of irrationalism?

Our age, which is so sure and victoriously happy in its scientific sentiments, just as easily as an earlier overlooks the strength of the mystical urges carried over into the popular mind by various adventurers. It still stands at a loss before the riddle of anti-Semitism, which would seem to have nothing to aim at in this age of equality before the law, and which, in spite of this—perhaps even because of it—has a fascination even for the educated youth. Until now no one has asked for a professorship of anti-Semitism, but it is said that there are already anti-Semitic professors. Whoever knows the story of nature-philosophy in its most radical branches will not be astounded at such phenomena. The human spirit is only too much inclined to forsake the laborious way of orderly thought and lose itself in dreamy reveries. . . . One must learn and become accustomed to explain the unknown from the known, rather than, conversely, to choose the dark and unknown, as if it were a new truth, as a starting point in a search for fantastic conclusions.[39]

Virchow's Conception of Medicine

In 1849 Virchow wrote that he was a humanist and that humanism should be based on natural science and expressed in a fully developed anthropology.[40] Humanism was neither spiritualistic nor materialistic, neither egotistical nor sentimental, neither anarchistic nor communistic. It started from the individual person and recognized the right of every person to his own development. Virchow saw medicine both as one of the natural sciences and as the chief of the humanistic sciences. It was for this reason that his interests in medicine, public health, ethnology, anthropology, and politics were not, in his eyes, disparate. He summed up his attitude in the following statement:

Finally, let us recall the words of Descartes, who said that if it were at all possible to ennoble the human race, the means for this could be found only in medicine. In reality, if medicine is the science of the healthy as well as of the ill human being (which is what it ought to be), what other science is better suited to propose laws as the basis of the social structure, in order to make effective those which are inherent in man himself? Once medicine is established as anthropology, and once the interests of the privileged no longer determine the course of public events, the physiologist and the practitioner will be counted among the elder statesmen who support the social structure. Medicine is a social science in its very bone and marrow, as Herr Neumann, with the steely weapon of his sharp logic, points out in an essay on the relationship between public health and property—a work small in scope, but far richer in content than anything written in this field before his time. No physiologist or practitioner ought ever to forget that medicine unites in itself all knowledge of the laws which apply to the body and the mind. Schlosser is wrong when he attempts to show, in his history of the eighteenth century, that only belles-lettres and historical literature alter their physiognomy with political change; it is also wrong to believe that, in contrast to the political and religious sciences, the natural sciences can gaze into the deepest wellsprings of knowledge without feeling the desire to apply what they know. Let us recall the saying of Lord Bacon that knowledge is power, and be satisfied with nothing less from our great and promising science, of which Hippocrates once said: *Quae ad sapientiam requiruntur, in medicina insunt omnia.*[41]

It is all too clear today that Virchow's hopes were to remain unfulfilled. Medicine, far from developing into a humanistic discipline capable of adequately comprehending man, life, and disease, has become a technical craft working within a very narrow measure of the human being. It is not the medical man, but the lawyer, politician, or financier, who has become the "elder statesman" of our day. In the circumstance that Virchow's own efforts—though he himself came close to embodying his ideal—did much to further the special natural-scientific bias and limitation characteristic of modern medicine, we can discern an element of almost tragic irony.

Standpoints in Scientific Medicine

(1847)

WHEN WE SPEAK OF SCIENTIFIC MEDICINE, at the present time, it is highly necessary to reach agreement among ourselves concerning the meaning of the words.

According to our point of view it is self-evident that medicine involves the art of healing—although the most recent developments in medicine may make it appear as if this had hardly anything to do with the matter. Only those who regard healing as the ultimate goal of their efforts can, therefore, be designated as physicians.

Ever since we recognized that diseases are neither self-subsistent, circumscribed, autonomous organisms, nor entities which have forced their way into the body, nor parasites rooted on it, but that they represent only the course of physiological phenomena under altered conditions—ever since this time the goal of therapy has had to be the maintenance or the reestablishment of normal physiological conditions.

The actual accomplishment or, put more precisely, the striving for an actual accomplishment, of this aim comprises the task of practical medicine.

Scientific medicine, for its part, has as its object the investigation of those altered conditions which characterize the diseased body or various ailing organs, the identification of abnormalities in the phenomena of life as they occur under specifically altered conditions, and, finally, the discovery of means for abolishing these abnormal conditions. It presupposes therefore a knowledge of the normal course of the phenomena of life and the conditions under which this course is possible. It is therefore based on physiology. Scientific medicine is compounded of two integrated parts—pathology, which delivers, or is supposed to deliver, information about altered conditions and altered physiological phenomena, and therapy, which seeks out the means of restoring or maintaining normal conditions.

Thus practical medicine is never the same thing as scientific medicine but rather, even in the hands of the greatest master, an application of it. The scientific practitioner, however, distinguishes himself from the *routinier* and the medical opportunist by making the achievements of scientific medicine his own, so that they form the basis of his performance and he serves neither the idol of accustomed routine nor that of chance.

Medicine presents itself to us in this aspect if we project an ideal picture of it. Let us not deceive ourselves into believing that the realization of this picture is not still far in the future. We know only in a very fragmentary fashion the conditions which determine the appearance of abnormal phenomena in the living organism, and even when we do know these conditions, often enough we do not, to our regret, know the means to eliminate them. Under such circumstances the practical physician has the right to cherish a certain degree of empiricism, but so much the greater is his obligation to abolish this empiricism by means of his own observations and to help in the raising of the glorious structure of scientific medicine. The clinical physician is chiefly obligated because the clinic is the focus of medical practice. Hence the control of a clinic is such an extremely important matter at the present time, since the clinician of our day must be not only a scientific practitioner but an observer and investigator as well.

It is said that there are circumstances in which the split between scientific and practical medicine is so great that the learned physician can do nothing, while the practical physician knows nothing. Lord Bacon has said, *scientia est potentia*. Knowledge which is unable to support action is not genuine—and how unsure is activity without understanding! This split between science and practice is rather new; our century and our country have brought it into being. How could medicine go unscathed when an inner turmoil disrupted all relationships of German life? Who recognized a separation of medical science and medical practice at the time of Boerhaave and Haller? Yes, who knew at that time of a split between practical medicine and the entire immense field of natural science? But then there came years of deep spiritual oppression, a time of the greatest tribulation in the inner life of our people; in such a time it is granted only to the very great or very small among men to turn their eyes away from the immense changes in the body politic to the puny phenomena of eternal nature. French medicine has come out of the storms of the Revolution stronger and better than before, since the French people have actually completed a phase of their revolution. English medicine never broke the bond of science and practice, for the spirit of England moves steadily and undeviatingly along the appointed path. In Germany, at the time of the revolution, a philosophy was born, a philosophy which turned itself further and further away from nature, and a return to nature was possible only after this philosophy brought about its own dissolution. This return to nature manifested itself in the history of medicine in three stages: the stages of nature-philosophy, of natural history, and lastly, of natural science. Everyone knows the principles by which these three points of view have influenced medicine. The significance of each stage may best be assessed from the position which each assigns to hypothesis, since the three stages are characterized by a transition from an easygoing procedure to one less so, and culminate finally in a strict method. The school of the nature-philosophers, as is well known, based its medical system on its philosophy; to it logical hypothesizing was a completely justifiable equivalent for observation. The school which followed, calling itself very accurately the "natural-historical," partly absorbed this point of view during its development, and specifically it elevated proof by analogy to a position of extreme importance, exploiting everything from the whole of nature as it was understood, including past and present medical knowledge, and, with a great deal of spirit, erecting a structure whose supporting pillars were so many analogies and hypotheses. Medicine later reached the natural-scientific stage at a time when philosophy, too, had begun to turn itself toward nature and life; just as philosophy vindicated the old rights of the senses, so medicine threw off belief, cashiered the authorities, and relegated hypotheses to a housebroken existence. While used frequently enough in private, they are left at home when we step into the public forum. Both medicine and philosophy are in agreement that only a serious study of life and its phenomena can assure for them a place of significance. Only a precise understanding of the conditions of individual and community life will make it possible to establish the laws of medicine and philosophy as general laws of mankind, and only then will the saying *scientia est potentia* be fulfilled.

It is certain that scientific medicine as now constituted cannot permit itself to consider setting up a code of rules for medical practice, but is it therefore justifiable to retain a scientific and a practical standpoint in medicine? From the period of philosophical confusion we have clung to a conception which is nowhere further developed than in Germany and which has nowhere produced more harm than in medicine—I refer to the idea of "Science for its own sake," a detached science with its own goals, a science for the sake of mere knowing. This phrase recalls the nonhumanistic conception in which man regards his soul as the true reality, as his real essence, where he "knows himself only as spirit and has not yet come to value his corporeal part." True science possesses the ability to act, and it is a general law that everything which can be actualized desires to be actualized and strives for a real existence. Nothing, however, achieves real existence except as a part of life, and, just as the general philosophical viewpoint of the present day has thrown off its tendency toward the transcendental, so is the standpoint of a detached science devoid of effective force in medicine. It certainly does not detract from the dignity of science to come down off its pedestal and mingle with the people—and from the people science gains new strength. (Basically this "Science for its own sake" is only a piece of rhetoric. "Science in itself" is nothing, for it exists only in the human beings who are its bearers. "Science for its own sake" usually means nothing more than science for the sake of the people who happen to be pursuing it. If someone wishes to pursue science for his own purposes, if he has a need for knowledge, then the investigation and extension of his knowledge is the goal of his activity, and no one can object to this. If this man is a physician, however, and if he says that the healing art, be it in direct practical activity or in the theoretical elucidation of therapeutic measures and mechanisms, is the purpose of his activity, then it is self-evident that his science must include whatever is pertinent to this proclaimed purpose.)

To this desire for absolute science, although it indisputably brought great benefits for a while, we owe the fact that physiology has for decades remained foreign to medicine, and that medical observations have done without a physiological basis just as physiology has deprived itself of medical experience. Many a clinician, to be sure, has prided himself on his physiology, but often enough his physiology deviated in essential points from "the" physiology. There are bridges between physiology and practice, but few indeed have crossed over them, and the "physiological art of healing," one regrets, has not brought healing in its wake. In saying this no direct reproach is made against physiology; the greater portion of the guilt lies with the pathologists themselves, beating about with empty words year after year instead of providing themselves with definite concepts. They have had to suffer a good deal of misfortune because of this. Others came to work in their fields, and the pathologists rejoiced over this until they noticed that the seed yielded flowers but no fruit. Others, again, deposited eggs in the nest, which the pathologists, with a little luck, were supposed to hatch. Since they had, meanwhile, become somewhat mistrustful they were forced to swallow bitter parables.

Three times since the beginning of the natural-scientific period (therapy being entirely overlooked in these quarrels) pathology has suffered invasions which have left permanent destruction in their wake; once by chemistry, then by general anatomy and physiology, finally, and most recently, by general pathological anatomy. The result of these invasions is now, and perhaps will be to an even greater extent in the near future, a state of general confusion, an endless chaos from which the practical physician will issue forth with the greater mistrust the more often these upheavals are repeated. When he asks himself what of real value to him has resulted from all this, he finds, to his sorrow, little that he can use. Indeed, if the proponents of the movements in the field of pathology, among which open conflict has broken out, continue in the same way, we will soon have a group of self-sufficient, mutually exclusive systems of pathology.

It must be realized that now is not the time for systems, but the time for detail-investigations. There is a certain danger of a retrogression to crude empiricism in this procedure, but the danger is present only so long as an arbitrary attempt is made to draw general conclusions from detail-investigations. This is an error which the "systematic spirit of the Germans" has committed often enough; and it will disappear to the extent that the number of investigators, and hence the number of detail-investigations, increases. Let us seek general laws in the sum of these specific phenomena, but let us refrain from constructing systems which derive the phenomena from *a priori* general laws, or general laws from isolated phenomena. We have no use for systems until our experience is sufficiently inclusive to give us the guarantee that the system contains truth.

Chemistry has already accomplished a great deal for us, although thus far very little is useful for practical purposes. We expect a great deal more from it, but only if it devotes itself to individual phenomena more often, and places itself in the position of spokesman for medicine less often, than heretofore. We can learn much from chemistry, but we will have to reserve for ourselves the privilege of applying its findings.

General and developmental anatomy have given us much information about individual phenomena, but they can never give us a comprehension of the conditions determining these phenomena. These sciences, therefore, can never and will never participate in the real kernel of medicine, the art of healing. Pathology as well as therapy can be constructed only from within outward, and we dispute the right of any discipline not itself rooted in the contemplation of diseased life to share in the interpretation of its phenomena.

In this connection it appears to me that all those who understand the situation agree that pathological anatomy is the anteroom of medicine, and it would please me, least of all, to detract from its value. However, in the interest of pathological anatomy itself it appears to me advisable to elaborate on the value and significance of the subject for medicine, and to puncture certain extravagant hopes which have been founded on this discipline.

Often enough one hears the reproach that pathological anatomy has to do with end-stages but not with disease itself. Those who say this are half right and half wrong. It would amount to closing one's eyes before the facts of nature to deny that almost all diseases bring forth material, sense-perceptible changes in the body which of necessity belong to the history of the disease, and that the majority of diseases are accompanied from the beginning on by highly decisive, pathognomonic, material disturbances. To this extent, it is incorrect to doubt the significance of pathological anatomy in medical science. However, pathological anatomy has another side, and when this is considered, its opponents have a good deal of justification.

Let us consider for a moment the natural sciences in general, with respect to the mechanics of their development. Every natural science begins with a description of individual objects, more or less rapidly followed by their classification, to which, finally, the story of the origin and development of these objects is added. The descriptive part is only propaedeutic and its greatest achievements can have no more than an aesthetic interest; it is thus that we learn to know the properties of things, without learning of their interrelationships. Classification is a requirement of the ordering intellect; though it can be scientific to a high degree, its significance is nevertheless purely practical; it is used for scientific orientation and mutual, effortless communication. Genuine science commences with the history of material bodies; it inquires into the mechanisms and circumstances of their origin and development, into the temporal and causal interrelationships between these bodies, being concerned less with bodies as such than with processes in them, that is, with phenomena and motion. This part of science can in general be designated physiological; the first two parts, anatomical.

Now in what manner does the scientific investigator build up the physiological part? Let us take one example. It had been known for a long time that all bodies possessed, to a certain degree, the property of heaviness; thus this was a general law. Newton saw an apple fall to the earth from a tree in consequence of this heaviness, and he asked himself why the apple did not fall toward the sky. Investigating this question further, he discovered the new law that bodies were attracted along radii directed toward the center of the earth. Turning his attention to the heavens and seeing the phenomena of the earth repeated there on a grand scale, he discovered the still higher law describing the mutual attraction of the heavenly bodies—a law which has recently been confirmed, in one of the greatest triumphs of human assiduity, by the discovery of a new planet. Newton went further, however, and formulated a hypothesis which he could not prove, since the available facts were not sufficient for this, the hypothesis of the existence of a mutual attraction between all matter. This hypothesis, a generalization of a proven law and a rational consequence of this law, was itself elevated to the position of a law by the reflections of the following centuries.

Scientific investigation proceeds therefore in the following manner: a phenomenon of general occurrence is elevated to the position of a law, and when this law is applied to things which have not yet been discovered, a hypothesis is set up. Evidence is gathered for the proof—or better, for the testing—of this hypothesis in order to find a new law. Hypothesis is thus an essential part of scientific investigation, for it represents the thinking which must precede every rational action. To an equal degree analogy belongs to scientific investigation, for it is precisely by the drawing of analogies that the generalization of a known law to form a new hypothesis is carried out. The hypotheses and analogies in themselves have no value in scientific investigation except to the extent that they function as entering wedges for further investigation. The interest which our hypotheses have for us is thereby explained, for they are the growing and developing laws on which we test our strength, while the already discovered and firmly established facts belong to a past which every moment makes more alien to us.

Let us now take an example from the field of pathological anatomy. Cruveilhier[1] found it generally recognized that the loss of the lumen of inflamed veins in phlebitis was due to the presence of some kind of material of firm, semi-firm, or soft consistency. Thus this was a rule of pathological anatomy. Through his own investigations Cruveilhier further discovered that a blood clot could be found in the lumen prior to the appearance of any kind of change in the venous wall. This constituted a new and more definite regularity. The question then arose: How did the blood come to clot at this particular site? Cruveilhier carried his investigations no further but, with the aid of a hypothesis and a combination of findings, derived the more general rule that the first result of venous inflammation was the coagulation of venous blood. From this a new question resulted: In what way did inflammation bring about the coagulation of venous blood? Cruveilhier did not investigate this point either, but, with the aid of a new hypothesis and a new combination of findings, derived a third and most general rule: that the inflammatory process consisted wholly in the coagulation of the venous blood within the lumen. Finally, out of the puzzlement over the occurrence of phlebitis in the large vessels, the conception of capillary phlebitis arose. In this state the question was handed over to the Austrian pathological anatomists. Now, in the investigation of infarcts associated with hemoptysis, which up to that time had been regarded as extravasates in the lung parenchyma, Bochdalek[2] found that branches of the pulmonary artery were occasionally filled with blood clots and thereupon drew the following conclusion: since inflammation is equivalent to intravascular venous clotting, and, since in lung infarcts of the kind associated with hemoptysis clots are found in the pulmonary arteries, consequently this type of infarct represents an inflammation of the pulmonary arteries. It did not escape Bochdalek that occlusion of the pulmonary arteries by clots was at times not present, but since he had deduced the role from cases where clots were present, he could now say that this did not constitute a proof to the contrary since in such cases the inflammatory process occurred in the capillaries! Rokitansky[3] moved one step farther. Because of their peculiarity I want to give his own words: "Inflammation of the splenic pulp has not yet been demonstrated; the splenitis described in pathological anatomy is, according to its location, a phlebitis, i.e., an inflammation of the numerous intertwining and anastomosing venous channels of the spleen. One has, indeed, only to apply to a venous aggregate that which is known of venous inflammation (phlebitis) in order to derive a perfectly correct picture of inflammation in the spleen. The same thing which occurs in a simple blood vessel occurs there in a complicated arrangement of veins." Let us now listen to what has been taught about capillary phlebitis. "In the capillary system the demonstration of clotting in the vascular lumina involves many difficulties. It is evident that, in addition to the processes within the vessels and as a consequence of these, an exudation of serum and even of some plasma with blood pigment occurs. The vessels are obscured and made unrecognizable by this exudation. But, on account of the occurrence of the process in the great vessels, there ought to be hardly any doubt of its existence in the capillary vessels as well." The procedure of proof goes as follows: the spleen is an aggregate of venous channels, inflammation of venous channels is equivalent to coagulation of the blood, consequently inflammation of the spleen is equivalent to coagulation of the blood in the splenic vessels. This argument includes, in addition, a *petitio principii*.

Thus the method in pathological anatomy. What is the starting point for the pathological-anatomical proof of the existence of a capillary phlebitis? The fact that it is not known how blood comes to clot in large vessels. And why does the question of how phlebitis causes clotting arise? Because nobody considered that clotting of blood might bring about inflammation of the vein. In what way does pathological anatomy here differentiate itself from physics? In that pathological anatomy derives a law from a hypothesis, while physics derives a hypothesis from a law; so that pathological anatomy moves from hypothesis to hypothesis and physics moves from law to law.

Pathological anatomy in large part owes the great importance which it has assumed in modern times to ignorance, specifically to a complete lack of acquaintance with its history. Although care seems to have been taken to burn all historical bridges behind us, it seems only fair to the strict and just custom of German science, in particular, that they should be reconstructed. There is no longer a place for pathological anatomy as a dogmatic science; everyone must be clearly aware of the proofs for each law. But where to obtain proofs if the whole argument begins with a hypothesis? I could introduce many more similar instances, e.g. from the doctrine of crases; I will limit myself to the conclusion that pathological anatomy is really an anatomical science, not a physiological one, and that it can therefore make decisions concerning purely anatomical questions with the greatest of security, but concerning physiological questions only with great insecurity. Objects which we see only in their spatial relationships are supposed to be brought into a temporal and causal relationship. Is pathological anatomy able to do this in a precise scientific manner? In some instances, far more often than appears at first sight when the approach is made in a sufficiently unprejudiced manner, certainly; very frequently not at all. Although the most empirical and casuistic of all sciences, pathological anatomy as practiced up to the present time can only become a modern panegyrist of hypothesis. For how can one decide with certainty which of two coexistent phenomena is the cause and which the effect, whether one of them is the cause at all instead of both being effects of a third cause, or even whether both are effects of two entirely unrelated causes?

The final decision in these matters belongs to a science which at the present time exists only in rudiments and which appears destined to replace general pathology; I refer to pathological physiology. We define pathological physiology as the essential theoretical part of scientific medicine. "Theoretical" is obviously not the same as "hypothetical" since the former starts from observation and the latter from arbitrary decision. Pathological anatomy is the doctrine of deranged structure; pathological physiology is the doctrine of deranged function. It includes, therefore, pathological changes of the blood, the phenomena of abnormal circulation, respiration, nutrition, and secretion, the study of exudation and the metamorphoses which occur in it—in other words, the development of pathological processes—and finally, the study of altered muscle and nerve activity. It might seem as if all of this were very simple, as if one had merely to write out the laws of ordinary physiology and apply them to the several pathological processes. If physiology were complete, this might perhaps be correct; however, physiology, though a "respectable" science, is thus far a very incomplete one. When one asks detailed questions, one receives, often enough, a Delphic answer only. Physiology is not entirely responsible for this, since the detailed questions have hardly yet been placed before her by pathology.

What remains now to be done? The most comfortable and well-trodden way is to pass over such places with the aid of flying bridges of hypothesis and analogy. But if somebody follows behind with a more heavily laden wagon, the flimsy bridges collapse (if, indeed, they are still standing) and a state of sorry perplexity overcomes the leaders. It is for this reason that a pathological physiology is necessary, a physiology which does not stand before the gates of medicine but lives in its mansion, a science which knows exactly what medicine lacks, what investigations are required, and what questions need to be answered. Pathological physiology receives its questions in part from pathological anatomy, in part from practical medicine; it derives its answers partly from observation by the sickbed, to this extent being a division of the clinic, and partly from animal experiment. Experiment is the final and highest court of pathological physiology, for experiment alone is equally accessible to the entire world of medicine, and experiment alone shows the specific phenomenon in its dependency on specific conditions, for these conditions are arranged by choice.

A few examples will make my point clearer. In the course of the numerous investigations which have been devoted to diseases of the lungs in recent times, it appeared necessary and logically justifiable to search for the basis of certain pathological pulmonary processes in alterations of the circulatory apparatus. Now what could be learned from physiology about the circulation in the lungs? Physiology knew two things about it: first, that venous blood became arterial in the pulmonary capillaries, and second, that respiratory movements exercised a certain degree of influence over the movement of the blood. The first factor was itself without meaning for diseases of the organ; from the second, however, it was deduced that the origin of pneumonia was dependent on alterations in respiratory movements causing stasis of blood in the pulmonary artery and capillaries, and hence that to correct the condition required mechanical intervention in some measure. By means of a proof by analogy based on the behavior of the systematic arteries, pulmonary gangrene was construed to be dependent on the blockage of the pulmonary artery which had been observed in such cases. These deductions were just as arbitrary as they were characteristic of the hypothetical-philosophical method. The bronchial arteries were simply overlooked because the physiological textbooks no longer discussed such questions as whether the blood in the pulmonary artery had any function other than in connection with respiration, and whether the bronchial arteries sufficed to satisfy the entire nutritional requirements of the lungs. Now, as I engaged in experiments in the matter, it became obvious that a most extensive pneumonia could be produced by complete blockage of the pulmonary artery to one lobe and that pulmonary gangrene did not manifest itself as a result of this complete blockage. It was further shown that after two and one-half months of complete blockage atrophy did not occur. Instead, a collateral circulation developed which made a mockery of all accepted views about the development of collateral circulations. This circulation did not arise from the pulmonary arterial bed but from the aorta through the bronchial and intercostal arteries, occurring in exactly the same manner as had already been demonstrated after blockage of the pulmonary artery resulting from extensive destruction in tuberculosis; it was therefore possible to derive a general rule for pulmonary collateral circulation.

Another example: Saltpeter, it is said, has a beneficial effect on inflammations. Previously a cooling and moderating effect had been spoken of, something fundamentally related to the nervous system. The new humoral pathology, however, appeared to reject this point of view completely. Scientific therapy, for its part not satisfied with the simple empirical fact on very good grounds, had to have a more definite idea of the effect of saltpeter, but could demand from physiology no information at all concerning this point, for its investigation belonged to pathology, that is, to pathological physiology. Organic chemistry, which in recent years has moved so close to medicine, had meanwhile made a discovery well known to the older physicians, namely, that saltpeter dissolved clotted fibrous material. Now it was known from other investigations, themselves long known to the older physicians, that the fibrin content of the blood was increased in inflammation. To be sure, this was fluid, not clotted, fibrin. What could be more natural than that saltpeter taken internally made the fluid fibrin still more fluid, from which an extraordinary fluidity of the whole blood resulted! Whether the clotted fibrin of the exudate was actually dissolved by one or two drams of saltpeter which the patient took during the day was left still undecided. A short time ago Hertwig published experiments on animals according to which the use of nitrum internally *increases* the fibrin content of the blood. Saltpeter is thus again an empirical remedy.

Once again, therefore, let us not deceive ourselves about the present state of medicine! It is undeniable that our spirits are exhausted by the innumerable hypothetical systems which are constantly being thrown to the winds and replaced by new ones. A few more mishaps, however, and this time of disturbance will have passed by and it will be understood that only calm, industrious, and steady work, true work of observation or experiment, has permanent value. Pathological physiology will then gradually reach full fruition, not as the creation of a few overheated heads, but from the cooperation of many painstaking investigators; a pathological physiology which will be the stronghold of scientific medicine, where pathological anatomy and the clinic are only the outworks!

Scientific Method
and Therapeutic Standpoints

(1849)

WHEN WE RECALL THE APHORISM of the old Aesculapian—that
life is short and art is long—we marvel no longer at the eagerness
with which each man hurries to plumb the depths of the art in his
short span of life. And with how much pushing and shoving!
Millennia have passed over the heads of mankind, but no one yet
has grasped the secret of life. All have turned to dust before
solving the great riddle. Their gravestones proclaim the well-
known truth: *Ne quid nimis*. But who learns from the past? For
whom is there history? Who is born with the wisdom of his forebears? All in their turn have wanted to achieve everything, forgetting the lesson of the past that only in striving after a single,
consciously held, attainable goal, that only in building on the
firm and well-understood foundation laid down by our forebears,
that only in adapting to the almighty consciousness of our contemporaries, is there promise of great, secure, and lasting success.
All have begun by building a new temple and installing a new
idol. When those who were versed in history came to look, behold! nothing was new except the name of the builder. Every
system has attempted to anchor itself on the source of Being, on
that great Unknown which motivated the first impulse of Becoming against the resting Void. However, the experience of many
generations forces on us the realization that as yet no chain has
held. Still this mad striving after the infinite! And then suddenly in the midst of the commotion the implacable wave of an-

nihilation arrives, sparing the race but not the individual. The king, angrily insisting that no horny hand shall touch his golden crown, and the commoner, proudly standing on his good, inherited (though somewhat weakened) right not to be left to starve, are swept away. Many who look on this spectacle in terror might be able to learn—but care is taken that no one does. The very same people who cry out *memento mori* are only too ready to conceal its logical consequences. Heaven and hell have been invented and populated by these people in order to turn the eye of man away from the earth—that earth of his on which he has legitimate demands. To flatter his pride they bring up the old story that there is something divine in man—or, as others say, something demoniacal. But where is this inexpressible something to be found? Man watches the never-ending changes of appearance pass before his senses. Exhausted from the investigation of this eternal change, he, a creature of finitude, in his flesh subject to this ceaseless movement, a part of this movement and thus of the eternal, searches for the mid-point, for the source of movement in all Being. Then it is, they say, that the Divine emerges in him, and this Divine is supposed to be a part of the Prime Mover—in the Moved (which man is) a fragment of the Prime Mover is thought to lie. But the spirit of man, bound to matter and developing itself with the sense representations of this matter, can comprehend nothing which is not able to manifest itself in concrete material form. When man speculates about the original source of movement he is unable to transcend the sensual notion of opposing polarities. Hence, from time immemorial, philosophy has given prime importance to the polarity of spirit and matter, the opposition of different kinds of matter, and lastly, the contrarieties within the spirit. Medicine, always deficient in clarity of thought, has been satisfied to hypothesize a contrast of force and matter, an opposition of polarities, of cosmic and earthly influences, or the like. The Church, finally, since she does not recognize as fundamental the opposition between World and Deity, without further ado set up the Spirit, or Logos, as the origin—through Him all things were made, in Him was the life, and the life was the divine light of mankind. Revealed religion was logically the most consequent, since it postulated Spirit as something originally present without opposition—an incomprehensible statement of undenied transcendence, belief in which was compulsory. Philosophy and medicine, both resisting faith, either insisted that their own metaphysical statements were not really transcendent and their axioms not arbitrary, or demanded that their superficial conceptions (which were no more than tedious generalizations of poorly understood sense data) should be accepted as first principles. The natural-scientific viewpoint can no longer put up with the belief of the Church, with the transcendentals of philosophy, or with the platitudes of medicine; it recognizes the specifically human aspect of man as sovereign, and declares the earth to be the heaven of mankind. Unconcerned by the false accusation that this is self-worship or an apotheosis of egotism, or whatever else one wishes to call it, science takes the greatest pride in its own truth and freedom, and finds its most satisfying reward in achieving the greatest possible development of all the nobler abilities of man, whether they find expression through the muscles or the brain.

If we look about us at the present time, Europe appears to be filled with opposing camps. No proposal is without a champion, nor does any idea go unchallenged. It is as if this age of peace, denying itself in order to give birth to social reform, wanted to confirm the philosopher's paradox which states that development of *what is* occurs through negation. The natural sciences cannot idly stand aside in this battle. Medicine, aware of its sacred mission, dare not shrink away from the strife. Neither desk medicine nor medicine of the autopsy table, neither the medicine of reagents nor that of the stethoscope, will decide the outcome—it will be the physiologist and the practical doctor who will tip the scale with the weight of their experience. Every year brings us closer to the time of social decision. Let us see, then, what the banners of the various parties signify.

It is well known that, during the last three decades, intellectually aware German physicians have tried to rebuild the old bridge between medicine and the other natural sciences. All leading schools in Germany have agreed, and continue to agree, that medicine must be ranked as a natural science. It is the science of man, anthropology in the broadest sense, and—as an idealistic prophecy—it should be regarded as the supreme science. But when we inquire into the different schools we find their ideas about the implementation of this conception to be quite different. Let us therefore attempt first of all to understand how scientific work in general is pursued, in order to weigh the possibility of constructing a science of medicine, and in particular of therapy.

A year ago I attempted to point out to the society that the natural sciences are truly scientific only in their physiological aspects, i.e. those which are concerned not with bodies as such, but rather with processes, phenomena, and movements occurring in these bodies. The rest of natural science is merely preparatory. Physiology is the true natural science; everything else is descriptive or historical. I have further explained how the course of development of German medical science has passed, in a logical fashion, through the stages of natural philosophy and natural history to arrive finally at the stage of scientific investigation. I have indicated how these three stages really express no more than the transition from an incomplete to a complete method.

It is indeed true, as was emphasized by Asclepiades of Bithynia, the leader of the old school of methodologists, that it is the method of investigation which is essential and decisive. For what other reason has Lord Bacon become so worthy of the admiration of the ages—a man who (as James Fenimore Cooper cogently remarks) was a rascal, even though a philosopher? It was because he, for the first time with full understanding, after a long period of speculation, taught the scientific method, from which the natural sciences then quickly developed. It is a method which differentiates the Harveys, the Hallers, the Bells, the Magendies, and the Müllers[1] from their lesser contemporaries. This method is the spirit of the natural sciences.

The method of natural science, which, incidentally, is the only real method, since all others are merely procedures of exclusion, makes it possible to pose scientific questions. Everyone capable of properly posing such a question is an investigator. The scientific question is a logical hypothesis based on a known law, which moves forward with the aid of induction and analogy. Experiment, itself implicit in the question, gives the answer. A scientific hypothesis presupposes a comprehensive knowledge of the facts and is the outcome of a reckoning with them. Experimentation is a completely conscious and logically necessary action for a definite end. Anyone who knows the facts and is capable of logical thought can compel Nature to answer an experimental question, provided that he has the materials necessary for performing the experiment. Experimental investigation presupposes knowledge of the facts, logical thought, and appropriate apparatus. Methodically applied, these three generate the natural sciences.

All knowledge of facts is historical, not only because the facts are discovered by observations made prior to their application in newly arranged experiments, but also because one knows accurately only what one knows historically. The naked facts are doubtful weapons. It is necessary to know how they were tempered in order to estimate their strength. Medicine needs historical knowledge more than any other branch of science, and recent events have more than emphatically shown that the incredible present-day neglect of medical history will have its revenge. It is the unhappy privilege of Vienna to have conjured up a barbarism which has damned some of the newer schools to an undignified and murderous disrespect for tradition—schools which otherwise, on the shoulders of their forebears, could have developed a graceful and worldly air. Both history and daily experience teach that all knowledge is derived from the senses and that a law not verified by the evidence of our senses cannot be imposed on the human spirit for an indefinite time. Though an arbitrary law may have been upheld for centuries by force or casuistry, it may nevertheless be abolished at almost any moment. All progress rests solely and singly on the desire of the human race to penetrate ever more deeply, through ceaseless observation by the senses, into the eternal laws of its own nature and of the external world. Whatever one may say about Locke's sensualistic philosophy it cannot be denied that all of the newer movements in the State, in the Church, and in philosophy derive from him. Many were displeased, and still others declared that they were disappointed, when Alexander von Humboldt, in publishing his *Cosmos*, dispensed with a philosophical system. The investigator, however, knows only that which is accessible to scientific (sensualistic) investigation. How is it possible for him to describe the great Unknown when he does not directly perceive any of its qualities, and how can he deny it, since he is unable to prove its nonexistence? He knows that the wish to investigate or express something transcendental in comprehensible thought or words is, if not merely frivolous, certainly a completely hopeless venture. The conflicts between the Church and philosophy affect him only in so far as both occasionally invade his domain, yet guard against the prosecution of the consequences of his ideas over their Chinese walls into the realm of secular life.

The investigator knows only material bodies and properties of bodies. Whatever is beyond he calls transcendent, and he regards transcendence as an aberration of the human spirit. He understands material bodies and their properties only through the processes that occur in them. Since he becomes aware of bodies and their movements everywhere, since he is unable to conceive of anything, either in the past or in the future, except in terms of body and movement (his intellectual scope being formed, from the time of its earliest development on, as a resultant of the sensual awareness of these two factors), for him bodies, their movements, and matter in all of its contradictory manifestations, are eternal; when he talks of eternal forces he means the general laws of motion as products of opposites.

When the scientist talks about "life-force" he can mean nothing other than the resultant of that law of motion which presents itself to our senses as the formation of cells. For on this common ground both categories of the living, plant and animal, meet. This law is eternal, and everywhere made apparent, all-pervasive, manifesting itself where appropriate conditions are present. If we find no trace of organic life in the deeper layers of the earth's crust, while the more superficial layers harbor constantly changing varieties of plants and animals, this is in no way evidence for a later Biblical creation of plants and animals, nor for successive Divine legislation. We see in this only the fully comprehensible fact that cells cannot exist at a temperature of several hundreds of degrees, but instead carbon, hydrogen, oxygen, and nitrogen must form thick layers of gas about the glowing planet. Wherever we pursue the formation of cells, we find that it depends strictly on chemical and physical, i.e. mechanistic, conditions just as does every other movement found in nature. We conclude from this that cell formation must be a mechanical process just as is, for example, crystal formation. It cannot be said that cell formation is not mechanically determined simply because we are not yet able to express it in mechanical (that is, numerical and mathematical) terms, for with the same right an ignorant aborigine of New Holland would be entitled to say that a steam engine was not mechanically explicable. To argue in this manner is characteristic of the Church. Let us be on our guard and prevent it from spreading in the sciences, where there is dogmatism enough already.

As soon as the more highly organized animals pass through the earliest stages of cell division, we observe that the phenomena of movement are no longer limited to the formation and transformation of cells, but that tissues, organs, and systems of organs are developed with their own complicated, specific, and individual laws of movement. A currently neglected but quite justifiable distinction was made up to a few years ago between the motor and vegetative systems. Nervous phenomena were assigned to the former and assimilative, digestive, and nutritive phenomena to the latter. I consider this division to be as useful as it is justifiable, and from now on we will speak of movements in the nerves and movements of assimilation, digestion, and nutrition. When we observe these two kinds of movements in the mature animal, with particular reference to man, the question arises whether in either case there are things occurring which seem with any certainty to be determined by other than mechanical laws. As far as alimentation is concerned, it consists on the one hand in the mutual exchange of broken-down tissue constituents for new nutritive material through permeable membranes, therefore falling under the physical laws of diffusion, and on the other hand in progressive chemical alteration of substances in the body, from their intro-

duction to their removal. Although we are not yet able to explain
down to the minutest detail the physical or chemical processes
which occur, this is no reason for supposing that it will never be
possible to do so. Or should we, from our experience so far—
that wherever we have been able to carry through exact investigations, we have always been in a position to find a completely
mechanical explanation—draw the arrogant conclusion that at the
present time all mechanical processes are understood? It is a pity
that not a few people suppose that when processes are considered
as a whole something peculiar and individual always remains, and
that, for example, the process of digestion is inexplicable in its
entirety even though we are able to explain parts of it precisely.
In medicine such viewpoints are still countenanced, though it
would be rejected as preposterous if someone demanded of the
geologist that the precise history of every single acre of the earth's
crust be described; or if it were claimed that because every hill
and dale had not been specially studied, it was permissible to conclude that present-day notions of the formation of the earth's
crust were untenable; or, again, if someone said that the formation
of the earth's crust as a whole was inexplicable although the formation of every single layer was perfectly well understood. If
mechanistic explanations are desired in physiology, one must limit
oneself to simple processes and be satisfied to understand the few
things which have been carefully investigated rather than ask over
and over again "Why?" in circumstances where the human understanding has no starting point. "Mais Sa Majesté," said Leibniz
of the Queen of Prussia, "veut savoir le pourquoi du pourquoi!"
This importunate manner of asking questions, at once justifying
some kind of transcendence when no immediate answer is forth-
coming, has been, in all seriousness, directed toward the nervous
system. After a long period during which every manifestation
of nervous activity was regarded as something sublime, those who
held this view have been pushed farther and farther back by the
progress of our investigations. Since the relationships of the
nervous system to movement, sensation, and nutrition move closer
each year to an explanation in terms of known physical processes,
these people cling with the greatest of stubbornness to the unex-

plained relationship of the brain to psychic phenomena. Brain and psyche are dealt with by these doctors as were iron and magnetism by the old physicists. Should we not be satisfied with what observation has taught us up to the present time? In the nervous system we see two basically different constituents, ganglia and nerve fibers, that is, centers of stimulation and lines of transmission; although each of these two elements offers an array of varied phenomena, which we admittedly are not able to refer back to specific mechanical particulars, we see nevertheless a complicated web of arousal and transmission, of interlinkage and isolation, of inhibition and reinforcement, which complicates investigation to such a degree that a really unparalleled impertinence is committed when people who have themselves never lifted a little finger in the investigation of these difficult matters place before those tireless investigators who devote their lives to research the naïve question: "How then can the soul be explained from movements of constituents of the brain?" Can these gentry themselves explain how their personal psyche, their precious ego, manages to embody itself in matter? How their psyche stimulates the ganglia to activity so that a motor impulse arises to cause a muscle contraction? How the ganglia implore the soul to take cognizance of changes in the sensory organs?

> Connaissons-nous quel ressort invisible
> Rend la cervelle ou plus ou moins sensible?
> Connaissons-nous quels atomes divers
> Font l'esprit juste ou l'esprit de travers?
> Dans quels recoins de tissu cellulaire
> Sont les talents de Virgile ou d'Homère?
> Et quel levain, chargé d'un froid poison,
> Forme un Thersite, un Zoïle, un Fréron?
>
> —Voltaire, *La Pucelle*, Chant XXI

Let us leave these epigones of an intellectually surmounted though still influential epoch and content ourselves with the claim that mechanical laws have been met with everywhere, no matter how far we have pushed forward our knowledge of the human body. Even if we have met none where our investigations have been limited to the surface of things, nevertheless the time will come when we shall penetrate into the depths. If Columbus had believed the old wives' tales and held the New World for a fantasy only because he was unable to see its shores from the coast of the Old, if everyone after him had displayed the same sluggish spirit, the United States, that land of common sense, would not exist today. But it does exist, and even if all the lords of the Old World bury their heads in the ground like ostriches, the tidings of its existence will be transmitted to them through the earth itself.

I have believed it necessary to base the following observations concerning different standpoints in therapy on this broad foundation. Although others have perhaps said the same things more expertly, I believe I may be excused on the ground that they have found no application. It is possible for me now to be much more concise since the critical standards have been clearly outlined. You will forgive me, however, if in my presentation I limit myself to the situation in Germany.

It is well known that in this country we have reached the same conclusion—namely, that no genuine therapy exists—from two different starting points. As is evident, one side started from the standpoint of faith and the other from that of skepticism. In natural religion as well as in revealed religion it has been held since earliest times that illnesses are of divine origin, since otherwise the priests could have had nothing to do with them. However, from time to time it has been forgotten that from this the conclusion follows that healing is an act of divine intervention. (It is well known that in recent times the hand of the Bourbon King was considered to be a divine remedy for scrofulous children, an antiscrofulous power being attributed to the hand of the anointed King.) In our days in Catholic as well as in Protestant circles (although naturally with greater consequence on the part of the Catholics) this conclusion has again been called to mind. However, it did not please God to grant the blessings of success and long life to the efforts of Ringseis and Görres,[2] and, as far as the possibility of a Protestant priest-medicine is concerned, we have too much faith in the incorruptible power of the general intelligence to consider an advance attack necessary. Everything has its appointed time. A medicine of priests is only suitable for a people in the condition of childhood, and if medicine owes a great debt of thanks to the Christian Church (since it introduced, from Basilius the Great, Benedict of Nursia, and the order of the Knights Hospitalers on, not only the hospital system and the care of the destitute and ill, but also improvements in the science of medicine itself), nevertheless this service belongs to the past and can in no way justify a perpetual state of dependency of medicine on the Church. Our time is suitable neither for the Asclepiades and the Levites, nor for the Monks and the Deacons, and our medicine, like all useful arts and sciences, has put on simple civilian attire once and for all. If a poorly understood skepticism has simultaneously led to the same end, that of denying therapy, this can hardly be astounding to anyone who knows human beings and their history. Skepticism in people who do not have at the same time a special calling toward which to direct their attention has always given rise to confusion. When rumor includes even the honored name of Skoda[3] among the traducers of therapy, even then we cannot hesitate for a moment in expressing our concern over this trend. Yes, it appears as if here the neglect of medical literature, and the lack of any connection with the past of medicine (of which we have accused Vienna), begins to revenge itself. It is certain that many clinical teachers and practicing physicians do harm with the great number and frequent change of their medications, and that neither their judgment nor that of the older writers on treatment is trustworthy, or free from deception. Finally, almost nothing has happened in recent times to give therapy a firm basis. In spite of all this, however, we cannot permit the possibility of a useful therapeutic system to be everywhere denied, nor can disease be left to run its own course until the therapeutic Messiah appears, limiting ourselves in the meanwhile to diagnostic and prognostic studies. The statistical aggregates which have been assembled in order to test therapeutic agents can never yield results, since we deal with the treatment of individual sick people rather than of masses. If, instead of assembling tables, we had carefully kept up individual case histories, and physicians had worked carefully and circumspectly on the basis which a study of the older and the modern writers offers, then it would certainly have been possible to gather useful and convincing data. Only students and inexperienced practitioners are able to yield themselves up to an unrestricted praise of therapeutic skepticism. Everyday experience suffices to convince the unprejudiced practitioner of the effectiveness of therapeutic measures and medical activity. Certain things are so well understood by ordinary common sense and simple and individual observations that the most learned investigation, though accompanied by the endless heaping up of numbers, does not suffice to break down this insight.

Nevertheless, owing to the ever-increasing number of medicaments and a deficiency in the critical observation and study of their effects, doubt concerning their significance has by degrees grown so great that everyone who wants to accomplish something decisive for therapy in Germany applies himself to their investigation. The studies of Orfila[4] in toxicology, as well as the experiments carried out by Hahnemann[5] in the foundation of the homeopathic system, stimulated newer detailed investigations that—mainly since the discovery of the alkaloids—have taken on the peculiarly chemical characteristics through which they differ so basically from earlier work in pharmacology, which rested more or less on clinical observations. The unbelievably rapid development of chemistry in our century was certain to favor this tendency, the more so when chemists like Liebig[6] hazarded the attempt to participate directly in interpreting the effects of drugs. Thus a group of therapeutic explanations have gradually appeared in which one is aware of a lack of understanding of pathology— just as in the iatrochemical school of the seventeenth century, derived from alchemistry by pathologists, one notices a lack of security in chemistry—and, in particular, the erroneous principle that the physiological effects of drugs must first be known before passing on to the pathological has been generally accepted. In spite of the enormous and lasting approval that this principle has found, it clearly contains a most dangerous error, an error that has been a source of the skepticism mentioned above. Since knowledge of the effect of a drug is of interest in practice only in so far as it can be used in some type of disease, it therefore suffices for the practitioner to know that a specific effect follows administration of a drug in a specific pathological condition. The so-called "physiological school" of therapists supposes, however, that an explanation of this is required in medicine. Now it is a very justifiable, useful, and fundamental precept to think everything through to the end. The end of pure materia medica, of pharmacology in and for itself, is the beginning of therapy. But when will the end come? And is therapy supposed to stand still until then? This would again be quite like the Germans. However, as I emphasized a year ago, it should not be forgotten that pathology is not a mere transcription or application of physiological laws, as if when one or the other condition was altered by hypothesis the altered effect also could immediately be found by simple calculation. Therefore, no one can be allowed to claim that when we know the physiological effect of an agent such knowledge suffices for its practical application in disease. Does knowledge of the physiological effects of strychnine suffice, after all, for a knowledge of the manner, the diseases, and the amounts, in which it can be administered? In most cases we know only part of the physiological effect, and with this part we are as a rule unable to explain the pathological effect.

> Was man nicht weiss, das eben brauchte man,
> Und was man weiss, kann man nicht brauchen.

To keep to completely familiar remedies, can anyone, for example, satisfactorily explain the whole pathological significance of tartar emetic, calomel, quinine, and the balsams, from their physiological effects? People frequently behave as if they had a good grasp of matters when they acquire a passable understanding of the changes that a particular remedy undergoes in the bowel, or brings about in the intestinal epithelium, or even when they discover it again in the urine or sweat. No one will deny that such findings are very beautiful and well worth knowing, but what does the practitioner gain from the fact that iodine may be demonstrated in all secretions and excretions, that the salts of the plant acids pass out in the urine as carbonates, that a group of metallic salts undergo peculiar combinations with protein substances and reach the blood in such combinations? Does he thus know, perhaps, how iodine and the salts of metal and plant acids act? Or where he shall apply them? Certainly not. He can derive practical use from such findings to the extent that he can comprehend certain anomalies or differences in effect, and, according to circumstances, avoid or produce them. Thus, for example, he can understand why calomel gives rise to increased salivation at one time, and bilious diarrhea at another; he can alkalinize urine when it has excess acid that he desires to reduce, or avoid allowing the alkalinity to increase in urine already alkaline. Let us therefore not despise these efforts, but let us not suppose that they constitute the true path of therapy.

How easily the link with the chemical standpoint has everywhere been made! I shall only recall one of the most striking and at the same time most accessible examples of this kind, the treatment of chlorosis with iron, and I refer specifically to the statements concerning it made by Herr Carl Mitscherlich[7] in his lecture given at the celebration of the founding of the Friedrich Wilhelm Institute, on August 2, 1847. Herr Mitscherlich begins with a statement whose basis, it appears to me, is wanting—to wit, that completely developed chlorosis can be cured by no remedy other than iron; nevertheless, one notes that it is precisely in many cases of advanced chlorosis that iron is not tolerated, whereas many plant remedies exert a very favorable effect. Now when the quantity of blood cells increases with the simultaneous use of iron and protein substances, it does not follow that this increase must directly depend on the passage of iron-containing protein substances into the blood, since hematin, although iron-containing, is not a protein substance, and in the case of chlorosis the transfer into the blood of such an iron-containing substance has not been shown. One could just as well derive from this an increase in the growth of hair, which also contains iron. If in actuality "all symptoms of chlorosis depend on the altered blood"— which still remains to be proved—it is nevertheless certainly just as true that this alteration of the blood is not the real disease but

only the consequence of another kind of alteration, which we still
do not precisely understand. The formation not only of specific,
but of *all* cells of the blood is hindered—but how hindered? If
it were caused by a deficient intake of iron-containing protein substance, and if the formation of red blood cells depended essentially
on this intake, then we would probably have difficulty in finding
even a single case of chlorosis in young girls from the upper
classes, since they take a sufficient quantity of iron and protein
substances in their nourishment to form the necessary quantity
of hematin. At the highest reckoning it appears that up to four
ounces of hematin, containing two and one-quarter drams of iron,
can be found in the blood of the female. Now if one does not wish
to assume quite arbitrarily an extraordinarily rapid turnover of
this small quantity, then one must admit that a very insignificant
intake is necessary for its maintenance at the normal level. The
cause of chlorosis must, therefore, lie in some alteration of the
same relationships which determine the conditions of the normal
formation of blood cells and hematin; and if a normal digestion,
among other things, belongs among these, then every measure
which would bring back to normal the specific digestive change
(which we presuppose at this point, by hypothesis, in chlorosis)
would also have to be a therapeutic measure for chlorosis. No one
can deny that iron can bring about changes in digestion; therefore
its effect in chlorosis can be related to a change in digestion with
just as much right as to a change in the direct formation of blood
cells. Each of these explanations includes a hypothesis which up
to the present cannot be substantiated; the practicing physician
gains nothing from attaching himself to one or the other; it suffices for him to know under which circumstances he may hope
for success with iron in chlorosis; he has indeed the categorical
commitment to keep himself away from hypotheses whose wrong
application might easily cause harm. Quite similar considerations
occur in connection with the therapy of diabetes mellitus. Ever
since it was learned that the kidneys secrete only sugar already
present in the blood, and that all other organs of secretion do the
same, there have, in consequence, been repeated attempts to cut off
the source of the sugar—this to be achieved most completely, it

was hoped, with an exclusively nitrogen-containing diet. Now it is easy to see that dissolved sugar, like all other dissolved substances, must, and really does, pass from the digestive canal into the blood, and that the large quantity found in diabetes, or in mellitemia if you will, must be dependent either on improper formation of the chyme or on a failure of the sugar once having passed into the blood to undergo its customary changes. To hope *a priori* that one of these two possible disturbances might be eliminated by an exclusively nitrogen-containing diet is in any case somewhat utopian, particularly now, when the experiments of Bensch have shown that the milk of female dogs contains sugar even when the dogs are on exclusively meat diets.

Therefore, when I very gladly recognize the scientific seriousness of the efforts of the physiological pharmacologist and wish him great success, I must nevertheless state in opposition that this cannot be the shortest path to the foundation of *reliable* therapy, the present need for which no one will deny; I would even prefer to leave it an open question whether this is the shortest path to the foundation of *rational* therapy. These attempts to pilot "rational" pathology and therapy under full sail—"rational" signifying that which reasonably explains the phenomena—resemble the attempt of Icarus. Why explanations, when what is to be explained is lacking? Let us first determine what it is that remedies do in diseases, and we shall soon learn how they do it.

A reaction against this tendency could not fail to appear; and since on the one hand clinical teachers have made fewer and fewer communications of their experience at the sickbed, while on the other hand the possibility of therapeutic observations has been almost entirely done away with (particularly in Prussia as a result of the more than incomprehensible organization of the hospitals), it was certain that the reaction would originate among practicing physicians. The great success attained by Rademacher's work,[8] particularly in Prussia, and the enthusiastic manner in which even a new journal followed in his footsteps, should finally have brought an awareness to the government of the dangerous situation into which, as a result of its institutions, it had led scientific therapy. It is self-evident that the practicing physician and the clinician are the only ones who can assemble personal experiences with respect to therapy; everyone who does not stand by the sickbed can at best enunciate points of view, perhaps direct the investigation, and keep watch over the principles of therapy with a critical gaze—although in times favorable to therapy this, too, can be omitted. Accordingly, the clinician of the present day must definitely be a competent observer and not merely a teacher, and I most firmly reject the idea that at a time of such great therapeutic difficulty anyone can be chosen for a clinic on the basis of mere teaching ability. Not only the clinician but the practicing physician has a natural right, acquired if not inherent, to present his experience to the world and to consider it just as valid as the clinician does his; and I freely confess that in Rademacher's work I see the beginning of a reform that will end by rejecting the current "rational" or "physiological" standpoint in therapy in favor of the empirical standpoint. Only from this time on will therapy begin to develop like a natural science, for all natural science begins with empirical observation. Just as frankly, however, I must express my regret that matters had to reach such an extreme. Although Rademacher and his followers have quite justifiably adopted the empirical standpoint which had to be theirs, they have regrettably not understood how to raise themselves to the level of the natural-scientific method, in the absence of which a crude and pretentious empiricism, the consequences of which I have previously discussed, must in the end prevail. Let no practicing physician, therefore, hope for a therapeutic Messiah; let each one rather recall the proverb *Bist du Gottes Sohn, so hilf dir selber*, and this only after first making himself at home in the natural-scientific method. As we have seen, this method presupposes an extended knowledge of the facts, and here we particularly include the continuous progress in diagnosis and prognosis generated by recent investigations into the nature and course of all kinds of disease-processes. A sure development of therapy is only possible in so far as relations are established with these investigations. Of what use can it be to hear that some remedy or other has abolished a disease of the liver or an inflammation of the lung, if there is no guarantee that liver disease was the essential difficulty, or that inflammation of the lung was really present? A most serious offense against logic and morality has been committed by those who have introduced into therapy a procedure to which they like to give the name of the "therapeutic experiment." A wager, not an experiment, is carried out when a sick person is given one remedy after another until the right one is found by accident. Could it be said that a person charged with extinguishing a fire was carrying out an experiment if he tried to put it out with an arbitrarily chosen group of fluids, among which oil, or perhaps alcohol, was to be found? When experimentation with such an object is desirable, a fire is ignited where it can cause no damage, or a fire is sought out whose possible continuation brings no harm to the property or safety of the individual or the larger community. The therapeutic experiment can therefore be carried out only on ill or experimentally diseased animals; in extreme cases it can be carried out on ill human beings where every known remedy has been exhausted—and even in such cases one still cannot act arbitrarily, or choose without very definite analogies. The testing of medications on healthy persons, of course, belongs in the realm of physiology, and therefore can for the present have only limited value in therapy. It seems to me that it is in no way justifiable to include the dangerous procedure of blood-letting here, as has been done recently; dogs are good enough for such experiments.

An attitude of despair toward therapy, due to the increasing neglect of the classical literature, to the failure of the clinical teachers, to the inaccessibility of the great hospitals, and, finally, to the misconceptions of the physiological, chemical, and rational therapeuticists, found particularly among many of the younger doctors, has spread more and more in recent years—this can no longer be denied—among the laity also. The uncertainty of the pharmacopeia and the lack of faith in medical skill are such current catchwords that hardly a novel seems to be written in which a physician does not play a deplorable role. A reaction could not fail to appear here also, but what else could have happened when the great majority of people were boundlessly ignorant of pathology? One group turns its hopes toward God, seeking protection in prayers, sacraments, and penances, in the belief that no further help is to be found in man. When this mood coincides with "purposes," the previously mentioned sacred or priestly medicine comes to the fore. The other group, believers also, though in a different fashion, throws itself into the arms of quacks of all kinds; the "metropolis of the intelligence" most richly nourishes this type of impostor, all the more so since they sometimes find powerful support. Finally, a third group, and this is really the so-called educated group, conjures up from its mind (unintelligent enough, at least in such matters), commonly with the aid of certain charlatans, an individual therapeutic system for itself, and usually finds then that a certain bodily remedy is quite specifically suited to it. By a very simple mental process it is then discovered that this remedy is suitable not only for other people but also for all possible diseases. As is well known, such remedies are found in all countries, and in recent times the Germans have only the merit of having preferred simple ones. I do not consider it necessary at this time to go into that history of universal remedies which reaches back into the most ancient times and will not end with mineral baths, water, ether, camphor, electricity, and gymnastics. In my opinion, the only check, apart from the slow progress of enlightenment, that can oppose this tendency, the only possibility of a lasting change in public opinion, can be found in a satisfactory revision of therapy from the empirical standpoint, and in a well-rounded and thorough education of physicians. The physician will then teach and help at the same time, and it will no longer be possible for hospital doctors and clinicians to remain unaware of a therapeutic technique such as hydrotherapy, practiced in its own great institutions and often with visible success, nor to fail to take steps toward evaluating the alleged successes of the hydrotherapists and making them accessible to science! For progress and the capacity to remain in the same state (*vis inertiae*) mutually exclude each other, in spite of the fact that one of the newer political parties has conferred the name of conservative-liberal on itself.

Far more logical than the hypothesis of universal remedies, and therefore much more cultivated by physicians, is, as everyone knows, the doctrine of specific remedies; it may even be said that no one who seriously considered disease and its treatment could allow the question of whether specific remedies exist for specific diseases to go unanswered or at least unconsidered. We have here the genuinely ontological standpoint in therapy, which corresponds to the approach to pathology that has so often been attacked since Broussais.[9] No one has more firmly held to this standpoint than Hahnemann and his followers. However, if one must in general assert of ontology what Lord Bolingbroke, a man as witty as he was unscrupulous, observed in his well-known letter to Pope—"thus is a thing bare and empty of all Being treated scientifically"—it must first of all be asserted of therapeutic ontology. As soon as one is convinced that disease-entities do not exist, one must also understand that therapeutic entities cannot be opposed to them, or, to speak in the style of Hahnemann, that a battle between two instances of the same entity cannot be engendered in the same body. This question has been adequately disposed of in scientific medicine. If disease is only an orderly manifestation of certain phenomena of life, normal in themselves, that occur under abnormal circumstances, with deviations which are merely quantitative, then all treatment must be directed essentially against the altered conditions; moreover, when, in the course of the same disease, together with a continual change of conditions determined in turn by reciprocal disturbances of new organs by those already diseased, new groups of symptoms appear and still other parts come under the influence of the altered conditions, then the therapeutic procedure must of course be appropriately altered. Thus a rational interpretation of specific remedies must concern itself only with the question of whether a definite, particular and specific therapeutic procedure—a therapeutic entity—ought to be set up for a definite phase of a disease.

With this question we reach the truly practical therapeutic standpoint, the real field of observation, the therapeutic battlefield. The question has therefore been already aired from all sides for a long time. Now an abortive, now an expectant, at one time an essential, at another a symptomatic, mode of treatment has been decided on, and the argument about this will not be settled for a long time to come. Let us seek only to establish a theoretical justification of these methods.

When a definite cause exists for the abnormal phenomena that present themselves in the unified picture of a disease, health can be restored by the removal of the cause, as long as the abnormal sequence of life-processes depends solely and singly on this cause. For example, when someone steps on a splinter and contracts tetanus, he can be cured by the removal of the splinter and the restitution of a simple wound, as long as a change has not been brought about in the nervous apparatus (owing to the immense increase in nerve impulses) capable of causing or supporting the phenomena of tetanus—a change that we can produce directly with strychnine. The therapeutic plan must therefore change to the same degree that conditions change, spatially or qualitatively. It is not sufficient to restore to normal the temperature of someone who has contracted pneumonia after a chill, for once a change due to the effect of cold on the nutritive process has been fixed in the walls of the air passages—a change characterized by alterations in the capillary circulation and the diffusion stream between the blood and the tissues—a new group of pathological factors appears, no longer having anything to do with cold. The presence of an obstructing mass in an air passage, deranged circulation due to congestion of pulmonary vessels with back pressure toward the heart, etc., a decrease in respiratory surface, an interference with expiratory movements, a change in the blood caused by the exudate and the respiratory disturbance, variously caused changes in the nerve centers—all these represent so many new things to be treated that with regard to them an ontological, specific, or essential method would be a mental aberration. It ought not to be overlooked, moreover, that even should remedies corresponding to many or all of the indications mentioned be discovered, the validity of therapeutic entities in no way follows. If, however, such remedies are actually found for the earlier stages of diseases—and the daily growth of experience shows that they do exist—then it is a categorical duty for every conscientious physician to use the abortive method. Knowledge of syphilis, scabies, and mucosal inflammations (blenorrhagias) gives the most valuable indication in this direction, and it is particularly unfortunate that the assertions of the hydropathists (frequently exaggerated, perhaps, but also certainly quite correct at times) concerning the treatment of other forms of inflammation, etc., still await careful testing by hospital physicians.

But if a more extensive scientific revision of therapy, with regard to its methods, is to take place, it becomes quite necessary for clinical medicine to make use of the experience of pathological physiology in another way than it has so far; specifically, it must become accustomed to a thorough analysis of the alterations grouped together under the heading of one disease. For example, there is continual complaint about the inadequacy of therapy in tuberculosis, yet pathological anatomy nonetheless demonstrates numerous and extensive foci of healing. But what is done to investigate the conditions of spontaneous healing? Hardly any attempt is being made to separate clinically the individual manifestations of tuberculosis (I do not refer to phthisis), the simultaneous bronchitic, pleuritic, and pneumonitic affections, the processes on the surfaces and in the walls of cavities, etc., and to deal with the treatment of these various factors. In most hospitals tuberculars are even regarded as undesirable persons!

These considerations will suffice to show that there is no absolute difference between the abortive and essential treatment on the one hand, and the expectant and symptomatic on the other, but only a relative difference in relation to the persistence of the disease and its sequelae. In the one case the disease is cut off quickly—throttled, as French therapy says—and the sequelae avoided; in the other it is permitted to take its course, it being granted the longest stage of convalescence, and the patient the longest stage of invalidism, possible. In either case, however, one alters the conditions under which a part, or almost the entire group, of physiological phenomena have been abnormally altered. But it will always be the task of therapy to find remedies that dispose of whole groups of factors at once, with one stroke, whenever possible; the limits of possibility within which such a method can be fruitful can already to some extent be inferred from our knowledge of pathological processes. Typhoid ulcers, lung cavities, and liver abscesses cannot be throttled, but there is no reason to doubt the possibility of throttling the primary processes whose outcome these conditions represent. Expectant and symptomatic methods of treatment can be properly admitted only for the end results of pathological processes. It is here that we may provoke the natural power of healing, a power with which we have no direct acquaintance, since we recognize no special force, but only a manifestation of general laws of development. It is precisely the expectant method, therefore, that will have the task of fitting in with the picture of spontaneous healing and its causes as depicted by pathological physiology, so that remedies with which such causes can be produced at will may be found.

Looking back over our discussion up to this point, it is our completely unprejudiced and impartial view that *therapy, cultivated from the empirical standpoint by practicing physicians and clinicians, will elevate itself to a science—which up to the present it is not—only through its union with pathological physiology.* Knowledge of the physiological effect of remedies, which will certainly always afford valuable leads, cannot at present form the basis of therapy, but by entering as a part of pathological physiology, it can serve only to help bind together practical experiences in a gradually developing scientific order. The theory of remedies, accordingly, will at some time cease to form a special scientific discipline; later it will be only a practical one.

Furthermore, as methods of treatment we recognize only two: one which effects either the direct removal of the disease-promoting factor (the greater part of surgery) or the abolition of whole groups of abnormal factors, bringing about a rapid end to the primary disease process (the abortive method); and a second which is concerned with the outcome of the disease, and strives to promote conditions for the appearance of spontaneous healing through the restoration of tissue, fibrosis, retrogression, etc. (the expectant method).

Certain viewpoints are common to both methods, however, and I wish to add something more concerning these. If what I say is not new, the fact that great and trustworthy practitioners have reached a similar conclusion can count as a guarantee for its correctness, and I am happy to be able once again to perform here the task which I have always set for myself, that of cultivating a bond with traditional medicine and of restoring this bond where it has been frivolously destroyed.

Particularly among younger physicians one frequently hears the question of what ought really to be treated, and indeed no clear answer to this question issues forth from the newer "rational" therapy. Traditional medicine distinguished *chiefly the disturbances of the nervous system and of nutritive processes*, aside from the so-called mechanical disturbances which were, of course, to be disposed of by mechanical means. I have already tried to show, in another place, that the old division of living phenomena into animal and vegetative, or into phenomena of the nerves and tissues (nutrition), is justified, and it is therefore quite fitting that I should permit this division to apply in pathology. In fact, when we consider pathological processes from a broad standpoint, we see, in addition to "mechanical" (i.e. macroscopic) changes, only alterations of nutrition (the products of which form the object of pathological anatomy) and alterations of nervous activity (the most important objects of clinical observation). Extraordinary as this may seem at first sight, it is nonetheless true. All changes in the muscles, for example, reduce to either altered nervous influence or altered nutrition; changes in the movements of the heart, the digestive canal, and the uterus may constitute particular objects of pathophysiological investigation and presentation, but in the end they fall into one or the other of these groups. All pathological phenomena of the vascular apparatus, again, reduce to changes in the cardiac and vascular nerves, to changes in the nutrition of the vascular walls and of the blood, or, if you will, of blood formation (hematosis). It might be objected to this that secretory changes should be dealt with separately, but, since we have above already comprehended nutrition in general as the expression of existing relationships between the blood and the tissues, a separate consideration of the secretions is not warranted. Accordingly, disregarding the "mechanical" disturbances, it can be said that the only objects of treatment are nutrition and nerve activity. It goes without saying that, in accordance with our conception of nature, we refer changes in nutrition and in the activity of nerves back to mechanistic disturbances as well, but since this expression is current for dislocations, fractures, obliterations, etc., we make use of it for the sake of brevity.

It appears, from a consideration of therapeutic experience, that in general the *nerves are treated in acute diseases and fevers, the nutritive processes in chronic and afebrile diseases.* Admittedly, this has not been clearly understood. We observe, for example, that the older physicians regulate their treatment of the greater number of cases according to the pulse—"the pulse is the barometer of disease." But the pulse is a function of the blood volume and the movement of the heart; the movements of the heart are dependent on the condition of the nervous system and the myocardium; the blood volume depends on the nutritional condition (since the blood is the focal point of nutrition) and on the capillary circulation (which can have a back effect on the volume of blood in the arteries); at one time it points to the constitution of the blood and at another to the diffusion between blood and tissues, in either case to nutritive relationships. The condition of the arterial walls is of slight worth in the observation of the pulse, but where it comes into account, here again the nutritive process or influence of the nerves is involved. Now, since the blood volume in acute diseases only rarely undergoes significant or, at least, lasting changes, the myocardium usually does not suffer; hence the pulse here chiefly indicates the state of the nervous system, which manifests itself in the frequency, rhythm, duration, and energy of the individual contractions of the heart. A large group of diseases is locally treatable, i.e. the nutritive state is treated; if it happens, however, that the diseases become generalized—as is said—and when the nervous centers also become involved, then general treatment (treatment of the nervous system) is added.

On more careful consideration it is found that *a large number of diseases only become dangerous when they come to involve the nervous system, while changes in the nutritive process are self-correcting.* Thus it suffices to interrupt attacks of malaria with quinine, although it is impossible to believe that the miasma (which, according to present conceptions, is taken up in the blood, and which has caused an alteration in the blood, as the great changes in the secretions suggest) is immediately eliminated by quinine; therefore it is necessary to suppose that only the sensitivity of the nervous system is decreased (cf. experience with quinine in rheumatism and typhoid), and that following this decrease in sensitivity (excitability) the remaining alterations are gradually and spontaneously done away with. We know that pneumonias are frequently self-curative under the simplest hygienic regime. But when we treat them, do we presuppose anything other than spontaneous cure? Do we still believe, perhaps, that we directly render the exudate chemically soluble and capable of resorption with our remedy? Certainly not. We limit ourselves in many cases to decreasing the bulk of the blood, which accumulates in certain locations (the right heart, the brain, the liver, etc.) owing to the disturbed circulation and respiration; we treat the nervous system according to the pulse, and we bring about those conditions under which, according to experience, endosmotic flow from the tissues to the blood is most easily and completely brought about. The most trustworthy teachers agree here that the amount of the exudate, its progress, etc., do not in general determine the plan of treatment. In delirium tremens the indication is not to restore the altered blood to normal, but to inhibit its effects on the brain and to decrease the excitability of the latter. It makes no difference how we achieve this, if only we do achieve it; the blood later corrects its defects spontaneously. Herr Munter and I have reported to this society[10] concerning our experiments with curare. We have shown that maintenance of the circulation by artificial respiration suffices to bypass the phase of the effect of the poison on the central nervous system, whereas otherwise the animals unfailingly die from paralysis of the respiratory muscles. If someone should say that we did not treat the nerve centers themselves here, nevertheless we gave them time to recover, and hindered the complete destruction of their activity which would otherwise have taken place.

These examples may suffice, although they could easily be multiplied. All such examples have one feature in common: they show that we are actually already accustomed to treating the nerves and letting the rest go. We had only been insufficiently aware of this.

Concerning the treatment of the nutritional state, I can be brief, since attempts to "revamp" nutrition are made every day by the therapists. There is no need of first mentioning that it is sometimes quite proper to consider the vegetative system as a whole—the nutrition of the entire body—as diseased, while at other times one is confronted by locally disturbed nutritive processes. It suffices, for the present, to have called attention once again to the two great groups (animal and vegetative) of phenomena manifested in ill persons, and it seems to us that a more exact study of these different groups might be enough to introduce some order into present therapeutic experience.

Finally, let us recall the words of Descartes, who said that if it were at all possible to ennoble the human race, the means for this could be found only in medicine. In reality, if medicine is the science of the healthy as well as of the ill human being (which is what it ought to be), what other science is better suited to propose laws as the basis of the social structure, in order to make effective those which are inherent in man himself? Once medicine is established as anthropology, and once the interests of the privileged no longer determine the course of public events, the physiologist and the practitioner will be counted among the elder statesmen who support the social structure. Medicine is a social science in its very bone and marrow, as Herr Neumann,[11] with the steely weapon of his sharp logic, points out in an essay on the relationship between public health and property—a work small in scope, but far richer in content than anything written in this field before his time. No physiologist or practitioner ought ever to forget that medicine unites in itself all knowledge of the laws which apply to the body and the mind. Schlosser is wrong when he attempts to show, in his history of the eighteenth century, that only belles-lettres and historical literature alter their physiognomy with political change; it is also wrong to believe that, in contrast to the political and religious sciences, the natural sciences can gaze into the deepest wellsprings of knowledge without feeling the desire to apply what they know. Let us recall the saying of Lord Bacon that knowledge is power, and be satisfied with nothing less from our great and promising science, of which Hippocrates once said: *Quae ad sapientiam requiruntur, in medicina insunt omnia.*

On Man

(1849)

Homo naturae minister et interpres tantum facit et intelligit,
quantum de naturae ordine re vel mente observaverit: nec
amplius scit aut potest.

—Lord Bacon

ALL HUMAN UNDERSTANDING is based on an awareness of the
relations of the individual person to what lies beyond him.

These relations become known as a result of changes excited
in the central nervous system by the sense organs.

Without the sense organs, without the transmission of changes
in the sense organs (brought about by relations to external things)
to the central brain apparatus, and finally, without consecutive
changes in the latter, in themselves and in combination, consciousness is absent, and hence intellectual activity is impossible: the
human being remains imbecilic.

The complexity of the relationships of the sense organs to the
external world, therefore, determines the extent of intellectual
activity and the scope of culture; without it the human being
remains simple and undeveloped. "Man is the product of his
environment."

Culture, however, consists not only in the scope of sensual
awareness, but essentially in the energy of the interrelated excitations of the central apparatus, in the communication of excitations
from the sensual receptors to numerous groups of ganglion cells.

Human pride has been pleased to set up in opposition to this
conduction of stimuli, a spontaneity of thought—the will—as
characteristic of the human species. The study of primitive peo-

ples, and of the individual human being from earliest infancy on, shows us that a primary spontaneity does not exist, but that from the very beginning only sensitivity or (unconscious) reflex activity—instinctive activity, as it is also called (*instinguo* from στίζω)—is present.

The newborn child still experiences himself as One. He sees only the changes in his central visual apparatus; he hears only the vibrations of his central auditory apparatus. Only through the simultaneous alteration of many sensual receptors, or through a certain sequence of changes in the same organ, does differentiation and distinctive activity come about.

By making such distinctions an understanding of the differences between external objects and interior changes in the brain, first brought forth through relations to external objects, a contrast between human being and environment, an awareness of the ego, gradually arises.

To the degree that this isolation by distinction progresses, the instinctive side of activity is lost and the original feeling of unity dissolves gradually into self-awareness, into a *dualism between I and not-I*.

Advanced science was once again able to establish the unity of consciousness when it demonstrated that the human being can only become aware of changes in his central nervous system, and that he achieves a knowledge of external things only after these have brought about changes in the central nervous system by means of the apparatus of the senses.

It follows from this that the human being has nothing beyond himself to comprehend (γνῶθι σαυτὸν), that everything beyond is transcendent for him.

Only egoism—the dualistic, i.e. the imperfect and unscientific, self-awareness—which has not yet made a breakthrough (although it has "eaten from the tree of knowledge"), could lead the human race to transcendence.

Transcendence has two paths: that of faith and that of anthropomorphism.

There can be no scientific dispute with respect to faith, for science and faith exclude one another. Not that one makes the other impossible, or vice versa, but rather that belief has no place as far as science reaches, and may be first permitted to take root where science stops. If these boundaries are maintained, it cannot be denied that faith can have a real object. The task of science, therefore, is not to attack the objects of faith, but to establish the limits beyond which knowledge cannot go and to found a unified self-consciousness within these limits.

Anthropomorphism is an attempt on the part of the dualistic consciousness to return to the original unity. The path of this anabasis, that of analogy, is the path invariably trodden by the unscientific.

Religious anthropomorphism puts forward a God who resembles man, philosophical anthropomorphism the illimitable character of human thought.

Once one touches on transcendental questions, once one attempts to overstep the boundaries of self-knowledge, nothing else is possible. Since the human being possesses in his consciousness only the possibility of knowing the changes in his own brain, nothing further remains to him than to potentiate his own qualities unendingly. The qualities of the anthropomorphic God are only qualities—quantitatively elevated to the incomprehensible—of human beings striving toward a likeness to God, and human thought carried out to the remotest abstractions never reaches beyond itself.

The strivings of the dualistic consciousness toward unity, so long as they remain anthropomorphic, are thus immediately transformed into their opposites, after they have stopped for a moment on the dizzying heights of the Monstrous or in the formless vapor of pure Being. From the one the dualism of God and World arises, from the other the dualism of body and spirit, of force and matter, of being and non-being; in both instances in a transcendental, and therefore incomprehensible, manner.

The scientific consciousness, having achieved unity, does not need anthropomorphism, since it finds its satisfaction in humanism.

Rightly understood, humanism is not an apotheosis of humanity, since this also would be anthropomorphic, but scientific self-knowledge, arising from the complexity of the relations between the individual thinking human being and the ever-changing external world.

Its basis is natural science and its true expression anthropology.

Humanism, therefore, is neither atheistic nor pantheistic, for it knows only one formula for everything lying beyond the bounds of knowledge: I do not know. ("Natural science is modest"— Liebig.)

It is neither pure spiritualism nor pure materialism; constancy of force and constancy of matter are equivalent formulas for it, corresponding to its conviction of the *unity of the human being.*

It is neither egotistical nor sentimentally yielding, for since it recognizes the right of all individuals to unified individual development, it must necessarily ask for the same right.

Finally, it is neither anarchistic nor communistic, for since it proceeds from the complexities of natural phenomena and studies the law of the individual, it understands that the *complexity of individual existence, according to its inborn laws, is a necessity of nature.*

Cellular Pathology

(1855)

ON PRESENTING A NEW VOLUME of the Archives[1] to the public, the need arises anew for surveying the field of medicine and defining our standpoint more closely than before. It cannot be denied that we are gradually approaching a time when rival scientists (who at least are beginning to recognize themselves as such) will no longer completely split up science. We are becoming accustomed to scrutinize questions carefully, to pursue them methodically, and to seek no longer for answers lying beyond experience. This does not prevent personal conflicts, to be sure, but these are not without value for science. For we must appear in the arena, stand question and give answer, and seek for arguments and counter-arguments in experience; in all this there is practice in orderly investigation, in straightforward thinking, and in the drawing of limited conclusions. In a word, we are becoming accustomed to the scientific method.

If we return to the origins of these Archives—and this satisfaction will be permitted us—an extremely important advance becomes apparent. Those were days (1847) of great scientific degeneration in medicine. The method of orderly investigation had been almost completely lost. The great upheavals that microscopy, chemistry, and pathological anatomy had brought about were at first accompanied by the most dismal consequences. People found themselves helpless in the ruins as the old systems collapsed; filled with exaggerated expectations, they seized on any fragment which a bold speculator might choose to cast out. But one after another these fragments, too, valuable as they might be in themselves, proved useless; it was precisely what was expected of them that they failed to achieve, and in the end one hardly knew what to do with them. The reconstruction of medicine could not be carried out with fragments; what was so proclaimed turned out in the end to be a mere patchwork of formulas, a mirage without solidity or content.

Therefore, as the most important requirement of our program, we demanded the establishment of a stricter method. This involved the destruction of illusions by means of a pitiless critique, even at the risk of offending people. We declared war on formulas and demanded positive experience, to be gained to the greatest possible extent in an empirical manner with the aid of, and in the light of, the tools available. We asked for the emancipation of pathology and therapy from the oppression of the ancillary sciences, and we recognized as the sole means to this end the rejection of all medical systems, the destruction of medical sects, and the fight against medical dogmatism. We desired the authority of fact, the justification of the particular, and the rule of law.

Even at the present time it is surely very expedient to be reminded of this once again. For man too easily grows weary. Some have already had more than enough of the constantly new, of the heaping up of experience, and of the unceasing arrival of new workers. Time and again, systems are set up so that people may relax in comfort—for a formula relieves one not only of investigation, but in most cases of thought as well. First from one side and then from another it is proclaimed that there is now a sufficiency of facts, and that these should be put in order once again so that we may know where everything belongs.

On the whole, however, there is no doubt but that the better method has been widely disseminated; from the tumultuous state—which has not unjustly been called a revolution in medicine—of that period, the development of our science has followed a more even course, until now, as a result of the cooperation of an increasing number of workers, the prospect of better times seems assured. Many of the old troublemakers have penitently confessed and promised improvement; others have silently acquiesced and shown in their work that they are aware of the new trend. We know how to appreciate this, and although we have the conviction that only the younger generation, which has not made the flight out of Egypt with us, will be able to demonstrate the full significance of the recently accomplished reform, nevertheless, in the interest of the elder generation, it is still of decisive importance that the older authorities participate in the advance.

How much the Archives directly contributed to this situation is perhaps difficult to estimate. It cannot be denied the merits of having first unfurled the banner of a more critical movement, of having fought from the start against the exclusive efforts of the microscopists, chemists, and pathological anatomists, of having announced the independence of pathology and therapy with respect to the physiologists, and, finally, of having seriously persecuted rationalism and speculation. And even my personal opponents do not deny that if it has destroyed much that was considered high and worthy, it has laid firm foundations for much to come.

The tasks that the Archives will have to fulfill in the future are very simple. Above all else it will be necessary to add continually to the store of our experience. We cannot help those who shrink before the prospect of even more detail, for it is our conviction that we are only in the beginning of the new period. Just as the reforms of Paracelsus, Vesalius, and Harvey occupied centuries, present-day progress, too, will not cease within a few years. Our goal is the establishment of pathological physiology, and everything now available represents only a paltry fragment of what must yet be achieved. It is not yet a time for systems, and we can leave it to the day laborers and the coal barons of science to devise systems for those who need them. Just as civilization in new lands beyond the ocean was prepared for by vagabonds and robbers, so does science too need pioneers whose adventurous drives prevent them from taking part in the orderly work of true investigators.

However, we do not deny that it is desirable to achieve broad points of view, rather than to be overwhelmed by individual facts—and, moreover, by individual facts of restricted scope. The true investigator needs a point of view such that his investigations will not deviate too far from the common goal, just as does the busy practitioner, who is rarely able to apply an extensive critique to every new disclosure. More than ever this, too, will have to be one of the tasks of the Archives.

By and large, our feeling about the direction that must be followed is not only the same as our earlier one, but even more firmly seated. At that time we ended our article on the reform of pathological and therapeutic viewpoints by means of microscopic investigations with the following words: "It is necessary to advance our positions to the same degree that our visual facility has been extended by the microscope; all of medicine must move at least three hundred times closer to natural processes. Instead of working new discoveries into existing doctrinal schemes, we must found new schemes on the basis of these discoveries; on the other hand, however, previous experience, established over thousands of years, ought not to be thrown overboard. This, then, will be a true 'naturally growing' reform achieved by means of the microscope, a reform meeting all conceivable demands of clinic and practice, compensating them sufficiently for the fact that, in itself, *the microscope does not have the diagnostic significance ascribed to it by paltry and mistaken prejudice.*"

In spite of the widespread recognition that the microscope since that time has achieved, its influence has for the most part not yet penetrated. Only a few have advanced so far that they are really able to think microscopically, and it is just this that we ask. For most doctors, the older ones in particular, microscopy is like a foreign language in which they use the foreign words, to be sure, but think in their own tongue. For these people the microscope is a strange object that they use either out of curiosity and because it is fashionable, or for a definite purpose, namely diagnosis. And since fashion and curiosity are rather transitory, one is finally left with diagnosis as the sole practical viewpoint. The long and in part brilliant discussion that the Academy of Medicine in Paris conducted recently with respect to carcinoma and microscopy centered almost entirely on the degree of diagnostic reliability offered by microscopic investigation (or, more precisely, by the young school of Parisian micrographists).

As I declared a long time ago, in the passage cited above, the microscope does not possess the diagnostic value that has been attributed to it. I do not mean by this that it has little or no value in the establishment of a diagnosis. I am in agreement with Velpeau,[2] however, that it is not invariably necessary to enlist the aid of the microscope to determine that this or that tumor has this or that character. I, too, believe that without microscopic investigation I can make a reliable diagnosis of most superficial tumors. In general it is only necessary that each one gain for himself a sufficient measure of personal experience with the microscope. With most pathological objects one gradually acquires the habit of recognizing even with the naked eye how they would appear microscopically, for formation and regression follow a sequence of invariable laws that can be quickly understood. To be sure, there remain the more deeply situated or completely inaccessible tumors, in which, by means of exploratory puncture, one is able to take out small particles that can be better identified microscopically than by the naked eye. In this case, as Velpeau so neatly remarked, the microscope is an additional eye.

These individual instances can decide nothing with respect to the question of the general significance of the microscope. This can be assessed only in terms of the accomplishment of the microscope for the whole of science and pathology. For it must be understood that in addition to applied (diagnostic) microscopy, there is scientific microscopy, and that it is the latter which must finally determine the decision. What will in the end be of importance in the development of medicine is whether the microscope proves to be an agent merely of diagnosis or truly of reform.

Discussions of recent years have made it particularly clear how little trouble has been taken to reach the more general standpoint. Admittedly, the guilt lay on both sides. Practicing physicians and surgeons too rarely took up the task of following the course of disease processes with more delicate tools, and anatomical, chemical, and physical specialists customarily spared themselves the labor of testing the value of their (often quite isolated) findings by means of experience in the observation of patients. Only too often, therefore, was there justification for the reproach that practice was unscientific (or at least only incompletely scientific) and, conversely, that so-called science was impractical. A few discouraged spirits have therefore drawn the conclusion that the newer science is altogether useless for clinical practice, and that the latter must continue on its own path; actually the only permissible conclusion is that the method of observation was imperfect, among the practitioners, the anatomists, and the chemists who busied themselves with the investigation of pathological processes.

A few years ago I had to debate this question with one of the most zealous investigators in German surgery. In a review of Schuh's book[3] I said: "Herr Schuh is himself not yet quite conscious of the real significance of chemical and microscopic investigations; often enough he mocks his own preoccupation with them, and not infrequently he considers the whole movement from a standpoint of mere curiosity. The newer methods of investigation have as yet no more than diagnostic value for him, and he has not grasped the fact that it is the task of our time to understand the physiology of these formations by means of genetic investigation. His physiology is still hardly to be distinguished from that of Richter and Walter, and in spite of his practical attitude one learns almost no therapy." In his new book Herr Schuh has sought to justify himself with respect to these reproaches by explaining that he was as little up to the task pointed out by me as was anyone else, and that he gladly left to others the saccharine practice of dreaming and the enjoyment of infallibility; meanwhile he, as a practical surgeon, stood on the same field of observation as his forebears had for centuries.

Now this sort of thing certainly accomplishes little. It is always a feeble defense for someone to try to excuse his deficiencies by assigning them elsewhere, or by ascribing to others even greater ones. That the field of observation, for the generation now alive, is still the same as it was centuries ago—even thousands of years ago—can hardly be regarded as a very new idea.

Und die Sonne Homers, siehe, sie lächelt auch uns.[4]

But under this old sun, and on this well-known field of observation, much has changed. A new group of instruments for observation has been placed at the disposal of the human senses, permitting the extortion of different answers from nature, answers that were heretofore beyond our ken, and at present what is essentially in question is whether anyone understands how to make methodical use of these tools. If someone has only an incomplete understanding of them, and if he does not have a reliable method, he remains just as lost on the old field of observation as were his grandfathers, who did not possess the more perfected tools of observation.

Whether someone is or is not a practitioner *ex professo* has little to do with the matter. Excision and cauterization offer no greater opportunity for acquiring knowledge to the one who carries them out than to the observer. Locomotive engineers would otherwise be more eminent as physicists than the scholars who make scientific observations on locomotives in action. Whether a tumor retrogresses, whether it forms metastases in inner organs, whether it destroys much or little, can be established in the most exact fashion as well by one whose hands were not directly involved in the operation. And yet this idea continually crops up. Herr Broca[5] in his monograph on cancer—hailed by the Academy in Paris—elaborated on this point in a most detailed manner, but in the end brought forth nothing of significance that the German reveries and dry academic learning so frequently taxed by him did not already teach.

If only people would finally stop finding points of disagreement in the personal characteristics and external circumstances of investigators! It does not matter at all whether someone is a professor of clinical medicine or of theoretical pathology, whether he is a practitioner or a hospital physician, if only he possesses material for observation. In addition, it is not of decisive significance whether he confronts an overwhelming or a modest amount of material, if only he understands how to exploit it. And to do this he must know what he wants and how he can achieve what he wants: in other words, he must be in a position to put the right questions and to find the right methods for answering them, as I have discussed in detail in my article on scientific method.

The practitioner wants the diagnosis first of all, and nothing can be said against this. When he considers tumors, for example, the question arises: How does he reach a diagnosis? What question should he ask? In our experience he asks first about the malignancy of the structure confronting him. But malignancy is nothing more than a property of certain kinds of tumors, and if we know we are dealing with a cancer, we know also that it is malignant. It is necessary therefore to know what a cancer is, and in what respects, leaving malignancy aside, it differs from other tumors. It does not suffice to say that because a cancer is malignant everything that is malignant must therefore be called a cancer, for this is purely circular reasoning. No matter how much people object, it is necessary to learn the different manifestations of tumors, in other words, their histology and physiology.

With all of his practical experience the busy surgeon, too, cannot in the end escape recourse to histology and the microscope if he wishes to achieve more than his predecessors. Surgery finds itself here in exactly the same position as, for instance, internal medicine is with respect to the techniques of physical diagnosis. The older clinicians, too, recognized their pneumonias and pleuritides, and many still with us even believe that they are better able to cure these diseases than the new disciples of percussion and auscultation. But who believes that everything they treated was precisely what they supposed it to be? And who does not have the conviction that many diseases were present precisely when their existence was unsuspected? How does all this boasting about practical experience help if we do not know exactly what we are dealing with? Certainly, if everything malignant has to be a cancer, and everything with a benign or moderately benign course absolutely cannot be cancer—when someone is ready with his conclusions before he has even started—then it is hardly worth the trouble of wasting any more words on the subject.

Unfortunately, things are not quite so simple. Herr Bennett,[6] who finds the world—in spite of his book on carcinomatous and carcinoma-like tumors—still in a state of confusion concerning the subject, arranged a short time ago for the Edinburgh Physiological Society to set up a special cancer committee, which was supposed to clarify the situation in a report. After this committee had sat for a long time, it finally dissolved without having reached mutually agreeable conclusions. Neither have the discussions of the Academy in Paris significantly advanced the matter. Why is this so? In my opinion, because matters have been too superficially conceived, and the heart of the question has not been touched; in particular we have not yet been able to free ourselves from the natural-historical standpoint. The classification of pathological end-results is still supposed to be set up according to the old example of natural-historical classifications, with certain specific properties being presupposed for these end-results.

Although I have already unburdened myself with respect to this point in my article "Specifics and Their Proponents,"[7] I will nevertheless make a few remarks in addition, since the importance of this subject has been insisted upon only too emphatically in recent disputes. Is there a basis for the assumption or presupposition that species differences, similar to those existing between different animals, also occur in the manifestations of disease? Cuvier[8] has very elegantly remarked that "Every organic creature forms a whole, a single closed system whose parts correspond to each other, and through reciprocal effects contribute to the same specific activity. None of these parts, therefore, can change without also changing other parts, and every single part, consequently, at the same time follows from and characterizes all others." Accordingly if, with the aid of this law of the mutual relationships of forms, every creature can be recognized from any fragment of any one of its parts, should it not then be expected also that every new formation may be diagnosed from any randomly chosen fragment of its elements? To this I answer No—not merely because experience speaks against it, but also because the conclusion is indeed quite false.

Since every creature represents an interconnected closed system, there is only one specific range of typical forms (or better, form-components) which it is able to produce. Whether it produces its form-components under favorable (physiological) or unfavorable (pathological) circumstances does not change the situation in the slightest. No unfavorable circumstance can do anything more than interfere with development, and thus pro-

duce arrest or deterioration in relatively immature form-components, or quantitatively increase development, although at the
cost of other functions and therefore to the detriment of the body
as a whole. However, I definitely deny that any pathological
process, i.e. any life-process taking place under unfavorable circumstances, is able to call forth qualitatively new formations lying
beyond the customary range of forms characteristic of the species.
*All pathological formations are either degenerations, transforma-
tions, or repetitions of typical physiological structures.*[9]

I do not know whether Herr Schuh will at this point accuse
me of dreaming or of infallibility. However, it is simply a matter
of fact, and I shall be quite willing to admit my error as soon as
counter-proofs are furnished, whether from medical practice or
from the armchair. If this should not be the case, and if the statement is accepted that pathological structures carry within themselves the physiological characteristics of the animal species in
which they occur, then indeed I can only repeat that the task of
our time is to pursue the physiology of pathological development
hand in hand with the stages of normal development. Whoever
does not feel himself capable of or called on to do this should
at least not measure the meager results of his investigations—
drawing smiles even from the originator—against what a better
method of investigation, or greater application with the same
tools, is able to accomplish.

Herr Schuh now believes that he has discovered the origin and
character of a group of neoplasms in the empty bubbles and
structureless vesicles of his well-known colleague in pathological
anatomy. In a third revision of the "Pseudoplasmen," the vesicles
of Herr Engel[10] with their interior spaces, nuclear membranes,
and outer coverings will perhaps find grace in his eyes. In combination with specific exudates this will generate a series of magnificent formulas. If only the current generation were not so averse
to dogmatism, and would let itself be put off with formulas!
Even the younger generation of the Viennese School can do little
with these empty bubbles and vesicles, and it is very praiseworthy
frankness, indeed, for Herr Heschl[11] to declare himself flatly
opposed to all this. At all events we must go back to what is pri-

mary and original if we want to understand development, and this primary thing is not the empty bubble, the villus, the papilla, the granulation, the wart, or whatever; *it is and remains the cell.*

No matter how we twist and turn, we shall eventually come back to the cell. The eternal merit of Schwann does not lie in his cell theory, which has occupied the foreground for so long and which perhaps soon will be given up, but in his description of the development of the various tissues, and in his demonstration that this development (hence all physiological activity) is in the end traceable back to the cell. Now if pathology is nothing but physiology with obstacles, and diseased life nothing but healthy life interfered with by all manner of external and internal influences, then pathology too must be referred back to the cell. This is the task that we have undertaken and pursued for a number of years in consequence of Schwann's findings—a task which in itself appears extremely clear and simple, yet which has achieved recognition only with the greatest difficulty.

My friend Lebert[12] will excuse me if I repeat here his statement, used more than once in his letters to me, that my pathology is the pathology of the future. This was often a consolation to me when it was declared on the other side that I wanted to lead pathology back into the Middle Ages, and that I was again bringing matters to light which had long since been put aside as done with. Both versions may be true, but I hope that they are true only within certain limits. The pathology of the past is not in all respects so contemptible as it may seem to many complacent spirits, and the pathology of the present is not so perfect that we may cease building for the future. To be sure, I have combated the humoral pathology of recent years—not without success, it seems to me—and attempted to bring the much despised solidary pathology to a place of honor again, not, as Herr Günsburg[13] insists, in order to develop solidary pathology once more or to suppress humoral pathology completely, but rather to unite both humoral pathology and solidary pathology in an empirically based cellular pathology. This, I confidently hope, will become the pathology of the future.

However, it is very much a matter of concern to me that this future be not too distant, and that our contemporaries rather than our progeny recognize what is valid in my movement. With regard to our younger colleagues I am much less concerned, since fortunately I have had abundant opportunity from the beginning of my public activity to exercise a direct influence on the development of their viewpoint. With the older group, however, the situation being what it is, this was true only to a very limited degree, and a meeting of minds is therefore particularly necessary here. Moreover, it is not altogether unjustly that they are startled when they hear that everything in pathology must ultimately be comprehended from the cellular standpoint, and it might easily appear that we no longer want to accept anything that has been observed only with the naked eye.

Now this is certainly not meant. Let us for a moment place ourselves in the situation of an astronomer. He is in every respect the converse of a biologist. As the microscope is to biology, so the telescope is to astronomy. What would we say today of an astronomer who did not understand how to use a telescope, or how could we in the first place call an astronomer someone who had not engaged in a most careful investigation of the heavens with the aid of his magnifying lens? Though we can see the sun, the moon, the stars, the Milky Way, and the nebulae with the naked eye, yet do we obtain even the faintest idea of the nature of these objects if we limit ourselves to observation with the naked eye? Does the astronomer not dissolve the universe of the heavens into a great number of telescopic pictures whenever he thinks astronomically? To the astronomer the moon, stars, and nebulae perceived by everyone are very different from what they are to the simple onlooker, who does well even to recognize the constellations.

With the tools of the biologist—and pathology is not the least branch of this beautiful science—everything that lives is dissolved into tiny elements, not all so small that their presence cannot be recognized with the naked eye, to be sure, but possessing a structure so fine that a clear understanding of it is completely impossible without microscopic study. In my article "Nutritional Units and Foci of Disease,"[14] I have shown that these tiny elements, the cells, are the actual loci of life and hence also of disease—the true bearers of vital function in plants and animals on whose existence life depends, and whose fine structure determines the vital expressions of living beings.

Life, therefore, does not reside in the fluids as such, but only in their cellular parts; it is necessary to exclude cell-free fluids (such as secretions and transudates) from the realm of the living, and intercellular material of cell-containing fluids (such as the *liquor sanguinis*, the much discussed blood plasma) as well. To the extent that cells, in contrast with pure fluids, still represent something solid, though in a very limited sense, we side with solidary pathology. But not everything that is solid can be looked on as a seat of life. Solid intercellular substances behave like the fluid intercellular substance of blood. It may be admitted that a trace of life-activity (left over from the cells from which and through which they originated) inheres in them, but no well-established fact indicates that this remainder is sufficient to maintain itself intact, or to carry on and transmit the life-process without the continual influence of cells. At most they can stimulate life-reactions in other tissues. My solidary pathology is, therefore, very restricted in comparison with that of the older school, and in no way does it exclude a refined form of humoral pathology, as Herr Seyfert[15] fears.

May we really hope to attract the present generation to such a biological conception? Does this new kind of vitalism not stand in irreconcilable opposition to the dominant tendencies of modern science? The condescension with which the proponents of chemical and physical viewpoints—even those who have only a very imperfect understanding of microscopic anatomy—look down on morphology is well known. And indeed, when one considers the great successes that have been achieved by the chemical and physical investigations of our contemporaries, one might well come to believe that nothing more can be done with the cell idea.

Such a thought is easily countered. Should it be possible to present life as a whole in terms of a mechanical result of known molecular forces—and this has admittedly not been done up to the present—it would not be possible to avoid designating with a special name the peculiarity of form in which the molecular forces manifest themselves, thus differentiating them from other expressions of these forces. Life will always remain something apart, even if we should find out that it is mechanically aroused and propagated down to the minutest detail. To no mortal is it granted to understand life in a diffuse, if you will, a spiritual, form—after the destruction of physical or chemical substance—and if this were really to happen, it would certainly be the worst blow that could be struck against the present-day scientific world-view. All of our experience indicates that life can manifest itself only in a concrete form, and that it is bound to certain substantial loci. These loci are cells and cell formations. But we are far from seeking the last and highest level of understanding in the morphology of these loci of life. Anatomy does not exclude physiology, but physiology certainly presupposes anatomy. The phenomena that the physiologist investigates occur in special organs with quite characteristic anatomical arrangements; the various morphological parts disclosed by the anatomist are the bearers of properties or, if you will, of forces probed by the physiologist; when the physiologist has established a law, whether through physical or chemical investigation, the anatomist can still proudly state: This is the structure in which the law becomes manifest. To whatever conceivable degree the phenomena of human life may proceed in a mechanical manner, the existence of the living human individual can never on this account be overlooked.

What the individual is on a large scale, the cell is on a small scale—perhaps to an even greater degree. The cell is the locus to which the action of mechanical matter is bound, and only within its limits can that power of action justifying the name of life be maintained. *But within this locus it is mechanical matter that is active—active according to physical and chemical laws.* In order to comprehend the essentially cellular phenomena of life we must understand the composition, the mechanical characteristics, and the functional changes of cell substance; as far as the course of investigation is concerned, there can be no disagreement regarding the fact that chemical and physical investigation is primary, and anatomical or morphological investigation secondary. For my own part it is hardly necessary to go into the matter further, since I have had, rather, to defend myself, from the time of my earliest writings up to the present day, against the reproach of having sought out too minute chemical differences.

Too easily, however, the question of the concrete significance of the thing toward which an investigation is aimed is forgotten in a quarrel over the degree of difficulty or accuracy of the investigation. It may be more difficult to isolate the individual substances composing a cell, or a body formed by cells, than to depict a cell or cell-structure, but the cell will always be higher and more important in spite of this. As little as inositol and creatin are more important than the heart in whose muscle they are found are they more significant than the individual, primary, muscle bundles. *The significance of the constituent parts will at all times be found only in the Whole.* If we advance to the last boundaries within which there remain elements with the character of totality or, if you will, of unity, we can go no farther than the cell. It is the final and constantly present link in the great chain of mutually subordinated structures composing the human body. I can only say that the cells are the vital elements from which the tissues, organs, systems, and the whole individual are composed. Beyond them there is nothing but change.

Accordingly, little as our conception opposes the mechanistic tendency, its opposition to exclusively humoral and solidary points of view—even the most modern—is great. As far as the former is concerned, the difference in principle is admittedly less prominent, for modern humoral pathology has never actually come to the point of developing the extremes of its position. As a logical consequence, the blood—held to be the central point of all pathology—would have had to be represented as the truly effective agent, but this view has never been directly expressed, as far as I know; instead, humoral pathology has stopped with the product, i.e. the exudate, without clarifying the agency or force forming the exudate from the blood, where it is considered to be already materially present. The Vienna School, therefore, although crasiological, does not culminate in a doctrine of crasias and dyscrasias, but rather in a doctrine of exudates; the opposition of our point of view to that of the Viennese has accordingly been most pointed on the subject of the doctrine of exudates. At present we are less concerned with following up this difference: consultation of the appropriate chapter of my Handbook[16] will quickly convince the reader of its magnitude. Briefly, the largest part of what is depicted in Vienna as a specific exudate derived from the blood is, according to my conception, directly derived from a parent tissue as a result of new growth.

The opposition of cellular pathology to modern solidary pathology (which, as is well known, has been everywhere merged with neural pathology) is far more obvious. In his new book Herr Spiess[17] has expressed it openly. His keen mind correctly concludes from my presentation that just as Reil[18] formerly claimed that the individual parts of the body were responsive to stimulation, so I claim responsiveness for all cells and cellular structures; and accordingly that I will not accept the limitation of irritability either to the muscles and nerves (with Haller) or to the nerves alone, along with the modern neural pathologists. However, he does me a great injustice when he depicts me as involved in a difference with Reil, since I am supposed to relate irritability to peculiar vital forces. When Herr Spiess says "But Reil correctly insisted that this irritability could only be based on the various forms and combinations of the individual parts," I miss here his usual acuteness of presentation. Not irritability itself, but only the varieties of its expression can be sought for in the morphological and chemical differences of individual parts. That a muscle contracts in response to the same stimulus which causes a gland to secrete can and must be ascribed to the differences of structure and finer composition existing between muscles and glands. That both parts are irritable, however, cannot be discovered in such differences, but rather in an inescapable similarity, present in spite of all of the differences. Herr Spiess finds this in nerves, I in the cells or cell-derivatives, among which, of course, I include the nerves. The feature common to the nerves is, as far as we know, an electrical substance; in cells we recognize nothing other than life, i.e. a movement transmitted from cell to cell, and bound to a nitrogen-containing or albuminous material. Since the electrical substance of nerves must likewise be thought of as in continual interior movement, transmitted from the time of the simple cellular (embryonal) period, the disagreement lies only in the fact than neural pathology desires to limit to the nerves what I ascribe to all cells.

It arouses the concern of Herr Spiess that I have permitted myself the expression "life-force," which I formerly avoided. I have never assumed "special vital forces," as Herr Spiess claims. I do not deny that this has its risks, though not so much on my account as on that of others who think of something quite different from my conception in connection with this word. In the end, however, a term is needed, and it would be impossible to find one that could not be misunderstood or misinterpreted. Nowhere have I even hinted that life-force is primary, or specifically different from the other natural forces; on the contrary, I have repeatedly and emphatically stated the likelihood of its mechanical origin. But it is high time that we give up the scientific prudery of regarding living processes as nothing more than the mechanical resultant of molecular forces inherent in the constitutive particles.

As little as a cannon ball is moved by a force from within, as little as the force with which it strikes other bodies is a simple resultant of properties of its own substance, as little as the celestial bodies move of their own accord, or as the power of their movements can be derived simply from their form and composition, so little are the phenomena of life to be fully explained from the properties of the substances making up the individual parts. That this is still done today is the last fruit of that obscure side of Hegel's philosophy (converted into orthodoxy by C. H. Schultz)[19] in which self-arousal of life was the supreme dogma. It is most peculiar that we have to combat just this dogma, which harmonizes so little with Church dogma. For *generatio equivoca*, particularly when it is conceived of as self-arousal, is downright heresy or devil's work, and when we, of all people, are the ones to defend an inheritance of generations in macroscopic forms, as well as the legitimate succession of cell forms, this is truly trustworthy testimony. I formulate the doctrine of pathological generation, and of neoplasia in the cellular pathological sense, in simple terms: *omnis cellula a cellula.*

I do not recognize any kind of life with respect to which a matrix or a mother-structure must not be sought for. One cell transmits the life-movement to another, and the force of this movement (possibly, or even probably, a very composite one) I call the life-force. That I am in no way inclined to personify this force, or to make it simple and isolable, I have already stated clearly enough. Here I may be permitted to refer again to my statement: "Since we seek life in the individual parts and attribute an essential independence to them (in spite of every dependency they have on each other), we can also seek only in these parts for the immediate basis of the activity through which they remain intact. This activity pertains to the molecular particles, with the properties or forces immanent in them, set in motion by the life-force, although we are not in a position either to recognize some additional interior or exterior power as effective, whether this is called a formative or a natural healing power, or to ascribe to the transmitted life-force some special activity (*spiritus rector*) other than the general stimulation of formative and nutritive movements."[20]

This quite sober viewpoint is far from being merely speculative; on the contrary it is so very empirical that I first broke through to it when I was able, by demonstrating the connective tissue cells and the cellular character of cartilage and bone, to divide the body of the adult vertebrate into cell territories such as were until then known only in the embryo and in many lower plants and animals. A unified view of the whole field of biology thereby became possible for the first time; moreover, a general principle—for which neural pathology has, up to the present, sought in vain—was found by combining different facts (therefore, by the speculative path). As far as the nerves are concerned, empirical proof that they possess an essentially trophic influence is lacking up to the present, but we can demonstrate empirically that cells possess both trophic and functional activity even in the absence of innervation. We must protest, however, when our remarks with respect to cells are interpreted as if they did not apply to the nerves. We have constantly emphasized that cells, whether isolated or growing together and developing into larger formations including nerves and muscles, are living and irritable. Nerves and muscles, however, even if more highly organized, nobler, and more important parts, are still only parts among other coordinated parts, each one of which can perform its peculiar task and can stimulate others to their own tasks. For not only do the nerves stimulate the characteristic functions of muscles and other parts, but in turn these other parts stimulate the function of the nerves.

There is therefore no danger that because of our numerous loci of life, we shall sacrifice the unity of the living organism. Admittedly, we are in no position to demonstrate unity in the sense of neural pathology. The *spiritus rector* is lacking; there is a democratic group of individual creatures with equal standing, although not equally endowed, held together because the individuals are dependent on one another, and because there are certain focal organizational points without whose integrity the necessary requirements of physiological nourishment cannot reach the individual parts. Every cell cannot fetch its nourishment from any distance whatsoever; most of them are dependent on their immediate environment, from which they extract more or less material according to the degree of affinity of their interior substance. Therefore, one can still say with Herr Spiess that the nutritive material must be "offered" to them, but it must be added that whether or not they wish to accept it depends on the cells; or, to speak less anthropomorphically, whether or not a cell absorbs material arriving in its environment into its own substance depends essentially on the vitality of the cell and the presence of a sufficiently great attraction between its substance and the environmental material. For the mere attraction between inner and outer substances does not, of course, suffice to explain the intake of the latter; materials could just as well be withdrawn from the interior of the cell to the outside in consequence of such an attraction, as certainly happens in metabolic processes. In a viable cell, accordingly, a certain quantity of substance must be present, less mobile or less subject to change, held together by internal attraction, and exerting resistance to the ordinary effects of external substances. The other substances undergoing greater interchange, increasing or decreasing according to the affinity-relation between interior and exterior, are probably deposited around this basic stock.

The nucleus and cell membranes show themselves to be the relatively permanent part of the cells; the cell contents are the more variable. When the former undergo essential changes the composition of the latter does not remain undisturbed. Growing parts sacrifice their functional capability to the degree that phenomena of division more clearly manifest themselves among the nuclei; a state of fatigue or weakness, necessarily indicating a change in the molecular state of the functional component of the cellular contents, then occurs. It follows, on the other hand, that the cell membrane is at different times more or less open to the passage of materials, that it permits various substances to pass through in a different fashion and is variably permeable to the same substances at different times. In a viable condition the red cell does not allow hematin to escape; when it remains in the same place, however, whether within or without a vessel, its membrane gradually becomes permeable to hematin even when the persistence of its elasticity cannot be doubted. As I have previously shown, one then observes a decolorization of the blood cell—the membrane becoming even more distinct and at the same time the surrounding fluids becoming colored. Just as little do external substances penetrate into the parts, as we best see in the case of the colored substances (madder, bile, pigment, etc.); specific parts have definite degrees of attraction for them.

At various places in my Handbook I have emphasized a matter which to me appears of very great significance for the understanding of these phenomena; I refer to the relation between function and nutrition. The best physiologists of the present day are much inclined to group both together, since it appears that function both determines and is dependent on nutrition, and conversely that function and nutrition lead to intrinsic changes in the molecular state of the parts. Correct as this is, nevertheless it seems to me that the essential difference lies in the fact that nutritive processes rest on the continued exchange of internal and external substances, while functional processes rest on alterations periodically taking place in the ordering and combination of substances already available within the cell. The functional processes cause new groupings of the constituent parts; the nutritive processes maintain the original groupings by exchanging the altered parts for new ones drawn in from the outside. Admittedly, there is one point where the borderline appears blurred—the phenomenon of tonus. In a previous paper I attempted to circumvent the difficulty by calling tonus a nutritive phenomenon in the pathological sense, contrary to the interpretation of those physiologists who regard tonus as a particular kind of function, or as nothing more than ordinary function. Pathologists (among whom, after all, the term originated) thought not necessarily of muscles alone in connection with tonus, but of all conceivable parts; atonia means not merely a weakening of contractile parts, but a loss of elasticity or a decrease of cohesiveness in general, of the cellular elements and of the intercellular substances as well. Tonus designates the normal degree of vital effectiveness of elements; this degree is dependent on the nutritive state of the elements, and is a preliminary condition of function; tonus represents the sum of those properties manifested in normally nourished parts in the absence of a special stimulus or arousal. Accordingly, muscular tonus can only apply to those phenomena that continually take place during the normal nutritional state of the muscle, whose intensity waxes and wanes with nutrition, while the degree of contraction stands primarily in relation to the greater or lesser intensity of the stimulus that the muscle receives from the outside. Atrophy and hypertrophy alter tonus under all circumstances; they do not directly affect function itself, but only its possible range.

Pure neural physiology, to be sure, attempts to assert that the nerves are the effective agents in all structures. Thus Eckhard[21] supposes that if muscle tonus really exists, it should manifest itself in such a manner that all muscles would be in a constant state of moderate contraction as long as they were in connection with a central organ through living nerves. However, in the vascular musculature, where it seems most feasible to consider tonus the cause of certain persisting states of contraction, we find regions where no nerves at all are known to be present, e.g. the umbilical cord, as I have often observed. Accordingly, one might suppose that we deal here with an intrinsic property of the muscle itself. But, as Eckhard states in another place, neural physiology understands muscle to be nothing but a substance that has been observed to contract after stimulation of the nerves leading to it; hence neural physiology does not pay any attention to substances in which contractions have been observed unless nerves have been seen to penetrate into and to activate these substances. He states further: "For the question at issue, ciliary movement, the so-called contractile substance of lower animals, the heart-anlage of embryos (as long as no effect through nerves on the heart substance is yet possible) and the like, do not fall within the scope of its consideration. All of these instances prove nothing more to the physiologist—in the most favorable case—than that movements occur in animal bodies independently of nervous systems, which is something that he does not deny."

Thus there are movements independent of the nervous system, and the question then arises whether these movements are bound to cellular elements. With respect to ciliary movement, this has been known for a long time; after I succeeded in finding chemical stimuli for this movement, one might have supposed that, here at least, irritability was bound up with cell substance. With respect to the so-called "sarcode," the contractile substance of lower animals, Leydig[22] has shown that it is contained in cells, in the hydra at least. Concerning the heart-anlage of embryos—recently made the object of numerous experiments by R. Wagner[23]—it has been definitely shown to be composed of cellular elements from which the future musculature of the heart is built up. Thus we can conclude that irritability at least in this region, as well as in the umbilical vessels, resides in certain cellular elements that do not, as far as we know, receive their impulse to activity from the nervous system.

All experiments and observations made on muscles actually supplied by nerves which speak for inherent irritability are set aside by "neural physiology" with the objection that the finest endings of the nerves might possibly have been active. Neural physiology has, to be sure, concerned itself very little with many matters, e.g. with the beautiful observations of Duchenne.[24] On the other hand, however, it cannot be denied that from the anatomical standpoint a gap in our observations is still present here. Moreover, it should be found out whether degeneration of the nerves can be followed into the muscles in all cases of paralysis. With respect to the acute paralyses, there is at best a high degree of probability. Thus, in experiments with Münter, I have shown that the red muscles of animals, with the exception of the heart, are paralyzed by curare, and Bernard found later that the irritability of the nerve is abrogated while that of the muscle persists—a combination of facts which at once very beautifully demonstrates the autonomy of cardiac contraction and the specific site of activity of the poison. But how can one counter the objection that some degree of irritability might still be present in the terminal nerve-endings, even under these circumstances? At this point, nothing more remains than to point out the old observation of the contractility of primary muscle fibers isolated under the microscope, rediscovered in recent years by C. H. Schultz.

Indeed, one would have hardly believed that so much significance could have been laid on the experimental demonstration of the locus of contractility in muscle substance. Once it is recognized that the locus of contractility is not in the nerve, and accordingly cannot be transmitted from the nerves to the muscle and must thus be inherent in the muscle, the only question which can then be raised is whether the muscle's characteristic ability to shorten itself can only be brought about by means of nerve tissue or whether there are additional ways of stimulation. Thus the irritability *per se* of muscle is not in question, but only the degree of its irritability. But if we find naturally occurring irritable structures whose muscular character is not in doubt, and whose connection with nerves is either unknown or highly unlikely (as is the case in the vessels of the cord, and in the heart-anlage of the embryo before the development of the cardiac nerves), then it is also to be concluded that muscular structures can be irritable in the absence of innervation; and one can then further assert, as the last and strictest, the requirement of "neural physiology" that every particular arrangement of muscles should be investigated to determine whether or not it is open to other than nervous stimuli. However, even without the fulfillment of this requirement, even if it should be shown that muscle of adult vertebrates responds with contraction to no stimulus other than one reaching it by way of a nerve, we can regard it as indubitable that the ability to shorten, i.e. contractility, rests on the peculiar structure of muscle substance (the "syntonin" of Lehmann).[25]

Neural pathology takes exactly the same position with respect to nutritional processes that neural physiology takes with respect to muscle function. It, too, does not admit lines of argument based on the existence of structures without nerves, but rather insists— very frequently presupposing a much wider distribution of nerves than has as yet been verified by observation—that nutrition without innervation is completely inadmissible. Here, however, we find ourselves in a much more fortunate position, since we can find firm support in the existence of anatomical territories, even in mature vertebrates, presenting clearly defined changes in the absence of a corresponding distribution of nerve fibers. In my article on parenchymatous inflammation[26] I demonstrated that we can trace the boundaries of disease to single cell-territories in the connective tissues, the bones, and the cornea, that is, in parts possessing nerves, and that we are even in a position to produce these localized diseases experimentally. When we put a very restricted part, comprising only a few cell-territories, of any type of tissue into a pathic (passive) condition by means of inflammatory stimuli (heat, caustics), there first occurs within this area a chain of active (reactive) changes, which very quickly proceeds, at a certain intensity of irritation, to the actual new-formation of tissue elements. The nuclei multiply, the cells begin to divide, and a neoplastic focus arises in the surrounding region, as has been known from gross observation, after all, for a long time.

Since it has been customary at this point to seek the help of an exudate ascribed to some special activity of the vessels—disregarding the fact that we have no conception of any such activity—our argument becomes extremely pertinent at sites where vessels are completely absent from the immediate environment of the lesion. Here I can only mention the center of the cornea once again, although neural pathology is not quite satisfied with this. But there are numerous other such sites. In particular I have emphasized the dermal papillae[27] which occasionally, as a result of local stimuli, show new-formations in extremely small foci in the absence of special branches of nerves or vessels corresponding to these isolated zones. In connection with the growth of chorionic villi, I have shown that the formation of new buds and branches begins with the budlike enlargement and protrusion of epithelium, and that a partial hyperplasia of the stroma follows only after the formation of epithelial buds. At such sites no nerves at all are found, and often no vessels either; the epithelial buds, rather, have to grow by the intake of maternal fluids, and their growth is therefore most luxuriant where the placental villi penetrate into the maternal vessels. Even in muscles one can observe nuclear proliferation in regions near pathological foci, with limits corresponding in no way to the well-known and often extremely sparse distribution of nerves, or to the particular arrangement of vessels.

In a word, the irritability of isolated individual cellular elements of tissues corresponds completely with the assumption of their vital autonomy, and, in particular, the process of new-formation of young tissue elements from preexisting parts takes place under circumstances similar to those holding for the cleavage and division of the egg under the influence of the sperm. Just as little as special innervation is demonstrable here, so would it be difficult to demonstrate it in pathological cytogenesis. That we do not come out with a completely universal innervation of parts cannot be overlooked, although, with a few limitations, I will not dispute this. In order to explain many particular features of the business of nutrition and formation, and at the same time to give reasons for the limitation of these particular events to very tiny structures, one would have to show that nerves possess not only an isolated influence on extremely small structures, but also that the same nerve could have qualitatively different effects, something which contradicts all previous experience. How is it possible to admit, along with Romberg,[28] that faulty innervation can bring about hypertrophy, tubercle formation, and cancer, when we know already that these products are qualitatively different and cannot be accommodated in the Procrustes bed of Henle's[29] hypertrophy? At this point nothing can be supposed except that the same element under the influence of different bodies performs differently, unlike muscle, which contracts more, less, or not at all.

Nothing has thus far been established by exact observation except that the paralysis of certain nerves is associated with a sequence of disturbances in the nutrition of certain tissues. No one has ever been able to deliver a positive proof that the stimulation of specific nerves increases the height of the nutritional process in the parts in connection with them, except indirectly through function. However, even with respect to the neuroparalytic disturbances of nutrition, it has not yet definitely been shown that the disturbance is a direct effect of paralysis of the nerve. The only observation which appears to speak for this is the well-known experiment of Magendie[30] and the pathological observations connected with it, according to which severance or paralysis of the fifth nerve causes an inflammatory softening of the cornea. Two circumstances are certainly worthy of note in this connection. First, there is the limitation of a more significant degree of nutritional disturbance to the cornea, although the fifth nerve does not innervate this region alone. Is it not in this case highly probable that nutrition is disturbed by certain unusual factors, factors under whose influence the cornea comes secondarily and only indirectly? The second circumstance which occurs to me, namely, the more active character of the process, also speaks in favor of this point of view. What happens here is not merely softening, or a kind of gangrene, but a genuine inflammatory process, ushered in by redness, swelling, cloudiness, exudation, and the formation of pus; this, therefore, implies irritation. If paralysis, that is, a lack of effect on part of the nerve, were supposed to excite an active increase in the intensity of the events of nutrition and formation, a state of complete confusion in our conception of the process would result. While paralysis of a nerve causes paralysis of the corresponding muscle as well, thus causing a deficiency, in the former case precisely the opposite would have to occur. Putting these objections together, it appears hardly a matter to be doubted that the empirical explanation for these facts, in themselves quite certain, has not yet been found. As in the case of the affliction of the lungs arising after severance of the vagi, where Traube[31] has found the irritating factor in the flow of saliva into the air passages, so an external irritant ought to be looked for in connection with the corneal affliction following paralysis of the trigeminal nerve. To be sure, A. von Graefe[32] has shown that neither simple removal of the eyelids nor simultaneous extirpation of the tear glands suffices to call forth similar lesions; however, the fact is that after the severance of the trigeminal nerve, in addition to dryness of the eye and protrusion of the bulb, abundant quantities of secretion and foreign material accumulate on the surface of the bulb, and that the animals do not remove this because of the insensitivity of the parts.

On the other hand, since it has been established that nerves do exert a very evident influence on the walls of arteries and veins in so far as these possess muscular elements, and that therefore, by paralyzing or stimulating these elements, they can bring about the most striking changes in luminal diameter, thereby increasing or decreasing the flow of blood to the various parts, one must guard against designating those changes that the nerves call forth in the tissues by influencing vessels as directly trophic changes. One should be less inclined to overestimate this influence in view of the fact that, according to experience, whereas a decreased blood flow has as a consequence a direct decrease of nutrition, an increased flow in no way causes a direct increase. For example, it is easily understandable that Schiff could follow the most striking kind of atrophy, especially in growing bones, after dividing the nerves, and I have tried to assemble a large group of such neural atrophies. However, it is not understandable that, after a similar division of nerves, a hypertrophy of bones should follow as a consequence of neural paralysis, as Schiff[33] believes he has shown. I have myself seen his preparations, and I am convinced that what has happened here is either a simple periosteal proliferation (the formation of osteophytes in periostitis), or actual necrosis with peripheral new-formation of bone; it seems to me hardly a matter of doubt that in such circumstances either the periosteum was directly damaged, or an inflammatory process extended from the wound to involve it.

Accordingly, after an unprejudiced probing of the facts, it becomes clear that a direct, active increase in the nutritional process cannot be traced back to increased innervation, as far as our experience goes. But neural pathologists might now, like the neural physiologists, argue further that we cannot be permitted to extrapolate experience derived from denervated parts to parts with intact nerves. To do this, it would first be necessary to discover some sure and unambiguous fact, such as is possessed by neural physiology in the case of contractions brought about by nerves. But as long as no such finding has been demonstrated, there is no factual basis at all for pursuing the question of the absolute dependence of nutrition on nerves. On the contrary, the indubitable fact presents itself that plants, lower animals, and many tissues from higher animals undergo active changes of nutrition as a result of the exciting or stimulating effect of certain external substances, changes which, at a certain intensity or quality of excitation or stimulation, go on into actual neoplasia. This is, as has been said in medicine for a long time, *the reaction of living parts*. Just as a muscle contracts under stimulation, so there occurs here a series of active processes, ranging from a mere increased intake of nutritive material to the division of nuclei and cells, i.e. to the proliferation of tissues. As a portion of a plant becomes larger when it is exposed to continued friction, damage, or persistent chemical irritation, e.g. an insect bite causing a tumor or gall, so does the effect of a mechanical, chemical, or any other kind of irritant cause enlargement, growth, and finally neoplasia.

Although nerves enjoy the quality of irritability, the capacity to be responsive, to the highest degree, this quality is not theirs alone. The peculiar softness and delicacy of their composition, rather, permits a reaction—or, to speak more precisely, an action—in response to stimuli which would not suffice to bring about significant changes in the arrangement of the constituent particles of other tissues. Hence conditions for the regulation of such disturbances are also much more favorable, and nervous phenomena much more frequently have a functional rather than a nutritive character. The situation is similar in muscles, although regulatory adjustments of the perfection seen in the nerves do not occur; specifically, the marked dispersion of disturbances which so readily takes place as a result of the great extent and many interconnections of nervous elements is hardly possible in the more isolated muscular elements.

Accordingly, if we ascribe the possibility of action in response to an external agency (external to the part in question only, of course) to all living parts, to nerves and muscles just as much as to simple cells and cell derivatives, we can also point out a certain distinction, the more precise designation of which is likely to be important. All living elements can undergo nutritive changes as a result of disturbances reaching them from the outside (never through self-stimulation); only a few (nerves, muscles, cilia, gland cells?) are in a position to manifest a more striking functional performance without significant nutritive change. If the latter phenomenon is designated *irritability*, in Haller's[34] sense, then the former can be distinguished as *excitability*, in the sense of traditional medicine.

Irritability, in the narrower sense of the word, is a quality limited to a rather small class of tissue elements, and it presupposes a particular and specific delicacy of intrinsic composition. *The capability of being stimulated, i.e. excitability in the broader sense, is, on the other hand, a general property of everything alive, and is bound to the cellular elements that are the true vital units.* Just as the physicist regards inertia, weight, expansibility, and compressibility as general properties of every kind of substance perceptible to the senses, so must the biologist extend to all living substance the ability to react to stimuli. However, since all life is bound up with the existence and development of cellular elements, the biological viewpoint must be based fundamentally on such elements. This can take place the more surely as these organic units lie within the bounds of sensual recognition, while physical atoms and molecules, the units of the physicist, can only be inferred from data gained by sensual observation; from a philosophical standpoint they are so little satisfactory that we can look on their recognition as nothing more than a provisory scientific conclusion.

When we require *cellular pathology to be the basis of the medical viewpoint*, a most concrete and quite empirical task is at stake, in which no *a priori* or arbitrary speculation is involved. All diseases are in the last analysis reducible to disturbances, either active or passive, of large or small groups of living units, whose functional capacity is altered in accordance with the state of their molecular composition and is thus dependent on physical and chemical changes of their contents. Physical and chemical investigation has a very great significance in this respect, and we can do no more than wish a prosperous development to the school which is striving to form itself.[35] But we should not conceal from ourselves that the story of metabolic interchange will be brought to a satisfactory conclusion only when it is carried back to the primary active parts; in other words, when it becomes possible to describe the particular role every tissue, and every pathologically altered part of a tissue, plays in that story. Therefore, although one may begin with the outworks, the ultimate goal, beyond the urine and the sweat and the various waste products of organic activity, must never be lost from sight, nor should it be supposed that these waste products are themselves the goal. There would always be the danger of suffering shipwreck in a more or less exclusively humoral pathology, if this were to be the case.

The practicing physician, however, once he has convinced himself of the finer construction of the body through his own observations, will easily become accustomed to interpreting his experience in accordance with this point of view, and, as I have said, will accustom himself to thinking microscopically. If the physicist, in accordance with his basic viewpoints, is able to interpret events as movements of molecules (which he has never seen, and will never see), the medical man is in a much more fortunate position. He has already accustomed himself, even more than is necessary and justifiable, to think and speak of capillaries and nerve fibers which he, likewise, is unable to trace with the naked eye! The task of our time is to develop and win acceptance for a point of view based on an understanding of the special peculiarities and interrelations of the different tissue elements; a point of view, accordingly, that is essentially specific, i.e. localizing, as I have previously pointed out. In this manner a really scientific and practically useful pathology can be achieved, and we, too, are convinced that this is the only way to the pathology of the future.

On the Mechanistic Interpretation

of Life

(1858)

WHEN, BEFORE SUCH AN ENLIGHTENED GATHERING, I attempt to deal with the question of the mechanistic interpretation of living processes, I must first of all allay the fear that I may be intending to renew those unattractive discussions devoted to the double-entry bookkeeping of the boundaries between knowledge and belief, which have so often formed the content of general lectures since the Göttingen session. Knowledge has no boundary other than ignorance, and I have the cheerful conviction that in Germany the Church will not again succeed in presiding as the arbiter of Science. A nation which shed its blood for freedom of conscience in the Thirty Years' War, and lawfully acquired it at the Peace of Westphalia, may be permitted to treat at least that question as settled.

Our task is of another kind. With the tremendous development of the natural sciences, empirical knowledge has by degrees so accumulated that it becomes extremely difficult for one person to maintain a general viewpoint; particularly in the biological disciplines we already see that their formerly very intimate connection with the whole of scientific investigation is greatly endangered. Nothing is more pressingly demanded than the reunion of former connections in our general knowledge, and the recovery of the full power of unity in mutual understanding. For investigators of nature at least should be united by a general conception of life. Either this is scientifically possible—and only then can biology, the study of life, be regarded as an object of methodical investigation—or it is not, in which case we must cease desiring to submit life-processes to natural law.

As recently as a generation ago, a certain unanimity was to be found in a conception of life which embraced all of nature. What great things nature-philosophy believed itself to utter, when it discoursed of a "life" of the atmosphere! Since it was known that the atmospheric ocean preserved with great constancy a definite mixture of distinct gases, nothing seemed more natural than that there dwelt in the atmosphere some specific principle, as in plants or animals, so that of itself its specific composition was maintained and preserved. But meteorology has solved the ancient riddle of whence the wind comes and whither it goes; it has found the conditions determining the movement of air in the changing relationship between sun and earth, and between one region and another; it knows that plants take up the carbon dioxide which animals expire, and, conversely, that plants liberate the oxygen which animals need for their respiration. Without plant and animal life there would be no stability in the composition of the air; in these, and these alone, life dwells. If one does not wish to sink back into confused and arbitrary reveries, the conception of life must be bound solely to living creatures. Plants, animals, and human beings are the only known carriers of life. Life is bound to these definite forms; the interpretation of the idea of life must follow from their analysis, and only that kind of interpretation which will be applicable to every form of life, be it so low or so high as you will, can suffice.

The problem of life in this more limited sense, therefore, belongs only to botany, zoology, physiology, and medicine. Astronomy no longer speaks of the life of stars, nor geology of the life of the earth. The heavenly bodies, however, also have histories, even if very little concerning these histories has been committed to writing. The origin and fate of the heavenly bodies is as yet inaccessible to observation, yet they show movement, activity, and development. The earth was not always what it is now, and with every moment it changes. But is it alive? Is there any kind of correspondence with the histories of plants or animals to be found in its history? Does it resemble us? What a perversion of the imagination would be involved in hatching out and nursing along such a notion! The earth has its like among other heavenly bodies, and it is just as little comparable with the living beings which it carries as it is with the ether which the conjecture of the physicist places between it and the other heavenly bodies.

Life does not manifest itself only in the generation of bodies leading a special existence separate from each other, maintaining themselves as such, and unfolding their activity through certain inborn powers. All of this applies equally well to the heavenly bodies, stones, and crystals. The special existence of the living is inalterably bound together with a specific form, in which both the basis of preservation and the direction of activity are marked out in advance, and which in addition displays phenomena of reproduction, regeneration, and multiplication unknown in all the rest of the world. By virtue of the specific form in which it manifests itself, every living thing has a special peculiarity and constancy of structure, and, within this structure again, a special peculiarity and constancy of composition and of inner arrangement. Only this correspondence of structure and composition gives us the right to group the lowest plants and the highest animals together in a single immense kingdom of the living, and to set this kingdom up in opposition to the still greater world of the non-living.

The *cell* is this peculiar and constant form of life. Whatever living being we may investigate, it always proves to be derived from a cell and to be composed or built up from cells. Plants present looser and animals closer-knit arrangements of cells, each one having certain characteristics in which they resemble others, or are, rather, precisely alike. It is not yet absolutely certain how few or how many characters each cell must unite in itself, or whether greater importance is to be attributed to one or another of its parts; it remains a point of dissension whether all tissues of the body at all times contain cell formations, and whether the lowest plants and animals possess cells in the full and generally accepted sense of the term. But the fact that cells are the customary points of origin, and the reproducers, of life, and that life has been essentially bound to them throughout its history, is no longer doubted. All branches of biology therefore find a common point in the cell doctrine; *the idea of the unity of life in all living things finds its concrete representation in the cell.* What had been sought for only in the realm of ideas has been found at last in reality; what to many appeared a dream has won a visible body and stands there truly before our eyes.

A peculiarly constructed nucleus, often provided in addition with a special nucleolus, surrounded by a more yielding mass condensed at the periphery to form a membranous boundary which is sometimes tough, sometimes delicate, all built up from nitrogen-containing proteinaceous material—this is the organic cell. In itself it is already complicated, and is an organism in miniature; in itself it is already capable of carrying on a separate existence as we see realized transiently in the animal egg cell and for longer periods in the lower plants. For the cell is either the living individual itself, or it contains, in outline at least, what we are accustomed to designate as such.

Life, however, beyond the generality and communality through which it is life at all, has something special and peculiar by virtue of which its varieties are distinguished. And these peculiarities and particularities are also to be found in the cells. The more developed the whole organism becomes as a creature, the more differentiated become the cells. In many algae the whole plant is still no more than a block of similarly formed cells arranged together. In the vertebrates and in man, only the cells of the same tissues or organs are like each other in the interior arrangements—the so-called similar parts guessed at by the ancients —while the cells of different tissues or organs show the greatest differences of inner configuration, and occasionally of outer configuration as well. This difference corresponds to the special activities and effects of the various tissues and organs; it explains the extraordinarily great manifold of capabilities of single parts of organisms and of organisms as wholes. From this we understand not only how generic or specific differences make their appearance in the various genera or species of plants and animals, but also how individual plants and animals within genera and species possess in addition certain individual peculiarities.

Cells give rise to the green of leaves, and to the marvelous glory of color in flowers, without thereby ceasing to remain cells. Likewise, cells determine all those different colors in feathers, hair, eyes, and blood, by means of which genus and species, race and variety, and finally even the individual, are so strikingly marked out. The business of respiration, which could not be provided for by the simple cells, is bound up with the green coloring matter of leaves and the red of blood. It is the cells which give rise to the rigid wood of trees and the freely movable mass of the muscles; the hardness of wood and the motive power of muscle vary not only according to genus and species but also according to the more or less favorable development of the individual. And thus analysis leads us upwards to the delicate structures of the nervous system, where sensitivity, motor regulation, and thinking, the highest distinguishing features of animal life, are bound to definite organized groups of cells. *Life is cell activity; its uniqueness is the uniqueness of the cell.* The cell is a concrete structure composed of definite chemical substances and built up according to a definite law. Its activity varies with the material which forms it and which it contains; its function changes, waxes and wanes, originates and disappears, with the alteration, accumulation, and diminution of this material. However, in its elements this material is no different from that of the inorganic, the non-living, world from which, rather, it continually replenishes itself, and into which it sinks back again after it has fulfilled its special purpose. Only the manner of its arrangement, the special grouping of the smallest particles, is peculiar, and even this is not so peculiar that it forms a contrast to the manner of arrangement or grouping exemplified in the chemistry of inorganic bodies. The kind of activity, the particular performance of the organic material, appears peculiar to us, yet it does not take place otherwise than the activity and performance of lifeless nature with which physics is familiar. The whole peculiarity is limited to the fact that a very great variety of material combinations is compressed in a very small space, that every cell is in itself the site of the most inter-related mutual influences, of the most manifold combinations of matter, and therefore that successes are obtained which occur in no other place in nature, since nowhere else is a similar intimacy of influence found.

As particular, as peculiar, and as much interiorized as life is, therefore, so little is it withdrawn from the rule of chemical and physical law. Rather does every new step on the path of knowl-edge lead us nearer to an understanding of the chemical and physical processes on whose course life rests. Every peculiarity of life finds its explanation in peculiar arrangements of an ana-tomical or chemical character, in peculiar configurations of mate-rial whose universally occurring properties and powers are ex-pressed in these configurations, though apparently quite other-wise than in the inorganic world. Even here, however, the differ-ence is only in appearance; the same kind of electrical process takes place in the nerve as in the telegraph line or the storm cloud; the living body generates its warmth through combustion just as warmth is generated in the oven; starch is transformed into sugar in the plant and animal just as it is in a factory. Here there is no opposition, only a peculiarity.

Thus the living cell is only an autonomous part in which known chemical substances, with their usual properties, are or-dered together in a particular manner and act in consonance with their ordering and properties. This activity cannot be other than mechanical. In vain has man attempted to find an opposition be-tween life and mechanics; all experience leads to the conclusion that life is a particular kind of movement of specific substances which, following appropriate stimuli or impulses, act according to an inner necessity. Every life-activity produces a change of the living parts; or, better, so long as the parts are still alive, their every change appears to us as an impulse toward activity and as a stimulus of a life-manifestation. When a muscle contracts, the smallest parts within it arrange themselves in a manner different from the condition brought about by rest, and at the same time chemical changes occur by which certain of these parts are de-stroyed or transformed. A muscle, however, does not contract of its own accord, and it is not itself the stimulus to inner change and activity; rather it receives a stimulus from the outside, and it cannot choose whether or not it will contract; contract it must when the external stimulus is great enough to disturb the quiescence of its interior parts. *The law of causality applies to organic nature as well.*

Is this not the purest materialism? This is the usual question now heard, a question already containing a judgment of condemnation. And how few even take the trouble to stay for an answer! As if it were obvious that the judgment must be condemnatory if the answer is in the affirmative! Is it not possible that experience, no matter how much it contradicts traditional prejudice, is nevertheless well founded, and might we not have far more right to demand the sacrifice of prejudice than to proclaim the damnation of experience? *In fact, however, the mechanistic interpretation of life is not materialism.* For what else can be meant by this word except the tendency to explain everything that exists and happens in terms of known matter? Materialism goes beyond experience; it applies the narrow standard of its knowledge to every phenomenon and it forms itself into a system.

Systems have great significance in natural science, but only when they are derived from experience. Most systems, however, are far more the products of speculation than of experience, for they bear in themselves a craving for universality, and they can satisfy this craving only by means of speculation. *For all empirical knowledge is incomplete and fragmentary.* Therefore a great dislike, and in many fields even a certain fear, of systems predominates in modern natural science; systems are admitted so that known objects can be ordered and classified, it is true, but only with the greatest discretion are they used as means of explanation. Fear of going beyond the boundaries of empirical knowledge is so widespread that even the writers most reproached for materialism resist the desire to make it into a system.

The mechanistic idea is so little materialistic that even religious presentations cannot dispense with it. The Mosaic writings say expressly, "And the Lord God made man out of a lump of clay and he breathed the breath of life in his nostrils," and that

He "formed a woman from a rib which he took from the man."
Yes, this picture of the earthly, mechanistic creation of man, man
who returns again to the dust from which he was taken, dominates
the religious doctrines transmitted to us to such an extent that
modern scientific investigation can hardly be reproached for being
to a greater degree mechanistic. Rather is its mechanism less
crude; it does not simply remain bound to rough general expressions, but, with the more advanced experience of our time, attempts to trace the context of the most minute events in all
creation.

Many people behave as if every ideal conception and all poetic
fragrance were thereby destroyed. The investigator who has left
all illusions of childhood behind is pitied; experience, no longer
limited to crude phenomena but penetrating into the inner essence
of things, is shied away from. It is supposed that the heart of the
natural scientist closes before the impressive spectacle of heaven
and earth; in vain does nature array herself in her most beautiful
colors, to no purpose does she appear in the most astounding
forms—color and form melt away before the indifferent eye of
the scientist, and he sees only material atoms moving without freedom and without meaning. Marveling only at itself and its vic-
tories, deifying itself, science has neither wonder nor reverence
now for greatness of another kind.

What confusion! One does not need to be a scientist to have
a cold heart and closed mind, or to harden oneself through self-
deification against every kind of humility before the merits of
others and against every impulse to admiration. From the philosophical schools of antiquity the stern admonition *nil admirari* has
already been transmitted to us! It is in the character and mood of
individual men, as well as in the education of the masses, that we
must seek the reason why individual men in the same eras, and
the masses in different eras, are inclined in varying degree to conceive of the world of phenomena now more figuratively, now
more objectively; why at different times persons behave in a more
emotional, a more calculating, a more poetical, or a more investigative fashion.

In earlier periods of the development of peoples, the voices of the gods themselves speak out of the thunderclouds, and the rainbow is a real bridge between heaven and earth; in our later time, the child, the more delicate woman, and the more enthusiastic poet may follow, with a hopeful or timorous look, the course of the "airy messengers," or descry in the formless mist all kinds of marvelous or familiar forms—apparitions or animals, human visages or distant mountains. Shall a self-composed man follow these dreamers? Must one always call on the supernatural for help, or yield to every trick of the unbridled fantasy in order to win from nature her charms?

Once again a comet stands in the heavens, more striking and brilliant than has been seen for a long time. Should we again regard it as a warning or as a threat to the sinful people, foretelling difficult times of war, famine, and pestilence? Or should we see in it only a joyful harbinger of a good vintage year? The heavens no longer have messengers to be sent out arbitrarily to serve one or another purpose. The astronomer is now able to reckon the path of the comet and to specify its orbital time. Some day it will return, and then return it must. Yet when the eyes of men shall once again tarry awhile in its observation, when another generation with perhaps a much broader basis of science looks forward to its appearance, should the flames of its mighty, fiery tail on the nightly horizon arouse less amazement? Should not the appearance of this wanderer out of the unknown even then arouse in the sensitive human being that sensation of thrilling wonder which every sight of greatness summons up in us?

No, scientific investigation does not blur the feeling for the beautiful, it does not weaken the impression of the sublime, it does not kill the piety that knowledge of the good and the purposeful arouses in us. The snowy crest of the mountains, the blue line of the hills, the rich green of the meadows, the rippling waves of the brook, the beauty of the flowers, do not fail to exercise their profound charm on our hearts. A longing for the pure enjoyment that comes from the peaceful contemplation of nature drives us, too, out of doors; our fantasy, too, is occupied with painting pictures of strange happenings, with conjuring up past and future events before us, with thinking up new forms and connections in the present.

However, our imagination needs no illusions. Why think of a Dryad in every tree, when we know from experience of a far richer life than the conception of a subordinate divinity would offer us? Why place Kobolds in the secret recesses of the cliffs, when the powers of stone, water, and air, the action and counter-action of warmth and of plant and animal life, reveal to us such immeasurably luxuriant pictures of activities? Is knowledge of the operation of law hostile to every feeling, to every emotional stimulus? Certainly not. On the contrary, it strengthens the stimulus, and only on our mood does it depend whether this stimulus is directed more toward the beautiful, the sublime, or the touching. The scientist does not require storms, comets, or extraordinary natural phenomena to arouse these feelings. Even the dull heavens of autumnal days, the diurnal rising and setting of the sun, the most ordinary and lowest processes of his own existence, offer him inexhaustible material not only for the under-standing but also for the emotions. And when the miracle loses the aspect of illusion, when it appears as no more than the mani-festation of natural law, is the law less to be wondered at? The miracle less worthy of astonishment? Can it really be believed that the human heart sacrifices a source of emotional stimulation when the delusion that a miracle is a unique occurrence arranged for a particular instance is destroyed? Is it not far more grip-ping to behold in the dazzling brilliance of the miracle the sudden revelation of natural law, a revelation otherwise concealed from our spirit behind the veil of mysteries?

Natural law is the miracle, and this law fulfills itself in a mechanistic manner on the path of causality and necessity. The cause has the necessary effect in its train, and this effect in turn becomes the cause of a new effect. One thing affects the other, be it in an ordinary or in an unusual manner—in either case it is equally to be wondered at. It is only that the unusual stimulates not merely our emotions but also our understanding to a greater degree, that it calls forth longer-lasting impressions and makes further demands on us when we attempt to comprehend it. But we comprehend it only in a mechanistic sequence of cause and effect. *For the human spirit is incapable of any other kind of comprehension.* It is pure delusion to believe that we have a choice among different paths. Neither philosophy nor religion can travel over other routes without reaching confused and arbitrary results that contradict the true essence of the human spirit. Up to the present time, every philosophy and every religion that has not accepted advances in knowledge, and has not solved the contradictions between tradition and experience in favor of the latter, has been transcended. The reform must be a permanent one, and just as the principles of the oldest philosophical and religious systems gained their form and content from the practical knowledge of the time, so must form and content yield to the progress of knowledge. The new always appears dangerous as long as it is new. The Roman Church itself has come to friendly terms with astronomy, and even the Moslem is no longer hostile to anatomy.

Admittedly, there is a place where the victory of the natural-scientific method will not be secure for a long time. Does the law of causality apply as well to the life of the mind? Is there not freedom here at least, although in other respects necessity reigns in the whole realm of nature? It is difficult to treat of a question where so much ill will, so many illusions, and such unnecessary involvement of the emotions confront the calm thinker, and where it is in addition so difficult to replace poor phrases by sober thoughts. What is freedom? Is it arbitrary action? Am I fully free when I do what I wish? Can I really make a choice, as human beings persuade themselves they can? Let anyone try it, and he will easily be convinced that he deceives himself. Freedom is not the option to act arbitrarily, but the capability to act reasonably. Mere arbitrary action is not free, for it stands under the dominion of the affects and passions. The truly free man, however, wins dominion over himself and his urges; he learns to offer resistance to his passions with the power of ethical principles. He disregards the action toward which his passions urge him; he does what his ethical sense or convictions dictate. In either case he is impelled; he finds himself always under the necessity of progressing from cause to effect. Freedom of action means nothing more than freedom of thinking, and this in turn does not signify arbitrary thought, but, on the contrary, thought taking place according to lawful necessity, where all obstacles are most nearly disposed of, where law manifests itself most clearly and beautifully. In the realm of ethics, too, the greatest miracle is only the simplest and the most direct manifestation of law.

Wherever we look, causality, necessity, and the rule of law! And yet some would set up the natural scientist as the enemy of idealism—he who seeks always after natural law, who everywhere opposes arbitrariness, chance, and wilfulness! Where has there ever been a philosophy more idealistic than modern natural science? Whence originate all these reproaches that we lack orientation toward the ideal? Let us not be deceived about this; all of these reproaches come from the camp of the spiritualists, whether they propose their spiritualism openly or in concealment.

There are also spiritualists among the investigators of nature, and it is easy to see why they seek to base their statements in the realm of organic life. However, it is certainly very characteristic that spiritualism, as a rule, only overcomes the scientific investigator when he approaches a realm of nature foreign to him. The chemist is not a spiritualist in chemical matters, but he is able to be one in philosophical matters, where he is a dilettante. For we cannot hide from ourselves that for every scientific investigator there are certain realms of natural science in which he is more or less a dilettante, and others in which he is a complete dilettante; and that at best his dilettantism differs from that of the ordinary layman only in that he is a master in at least one realm of nature.

Does the biologist find spiritualism necessary? One of the greatest chemists of our time has answered this question in the affirmative. He compares the living organism with a building completed according to a definite and previously determined plan. The architect carries out the plan down to the finest detail before the building is commenced; stones, wood, and all materials are then combined until the plan, with all its lines and relations, stands embodied before us. Is this not also true in the body as well? Is not formation here also accomplished according to a definite plan to which matter yields itself? Is it the matter which makes the plan?

At this point the questions quickly move beyond the bounds of experience; they become *transcendent*. The biologist first seeks for the plan, or, as we might otherwise say, for the law. The next question, then, after the law has been found, is how the law or plan is carried out, not who made it. Does the plan or the law contain in itself the means for its realization? Has it effective power, so that of itself it sets inert matter into motion, and forces it into organic form? Is the law itself the power, and has matter no other property than inertness? Every chemist will answer this question in the negative. Matter without properties and power is nothing; on the other hand, a law with power, a plan with its own effectiveness, is a substance. However one may try to resist, no matter how immaterial one may choose to consider this substance, it remains a substance. When this substance is supposed, as it is in living creatures, to give rise to the most manifold activities, and to carry out a very complicated mechanistic task, at this point it becomes a spirit, an organically arranged being, the *spiritus rector*.

The chemist has no hesitation about recognizing the *spiritus rector* as long as he is not in his own field. Within his field he is satisfied with the bare ideal law, and with matter possessing specific properties and powers. But does he not deceive himself about the difficulties? The chemical law in its purely ideal sense has no means in itself for control over matter; it has no mechanical power to perform the actual work. It is, rather, the chemical matter which operates, which is active according to its special peculiarities; the law is not outside of matter like an external Mover, but is entirely within.

Now let someone point out the difference between chemical and organic activity! Plant and animal bodies form themselves from chemical substances which unite with each other here as they do everywhere else, and the chemist would be the first to fight against the idea that the process at this point is other than chemical. Nowhere are the hands of the architect or his masons visible; the more closely we investigate, the more distinctly we see matter itself as productive and effective. Chemical bodies place themselves where they belong or they are pushed there by other bodies, but no foreign hand interferes in this finest of mechanisms except to disturb it. Everything foreign becomes a hindrance. The less disturbed the materials are in their gentle intercourse with each other, the more completely will the plan at last be embodied and the law realized. Thus, can the law be anywhere except within material substance?

It is a matter of complete indifference whether we consider organic or inorganic creation. There is no *spiritus rector*, no life-spirit, water-spirit, or fire-spirit to be recognized therein. Everywhere there is mechanistic process only, with the unbreakable necessity of cause and effect. The plan is in the body, the ideal in the real, the power in the material. There is no separation here other than in conception; in actuality both are found together, completely inseparable. The opposition between power and matter completely dissolves at this point, the plan and its execution merge, and whoever raises a question as to the Author of the plan must also, at the same time, attempt to seek out the Author of matter. In that event, however, it is not only the individual case that is involved, not only the various *spirits*, prime movers, and architects, one of whom permits human beings and another animals or plants to develop, or one of whom forms this, and the other that, particular human being. In such a case we no longer work with a question of natural science, which attempts only to understand processes in the given world and possesses no means to make the earliest origin of that world an object of investigation. Yes, it is then no longer a question of science that is involved, for no one knows anything of that which *was* before all existing things. Here is the boundary of the transcendent: whoever passes over it finds himself outside of the realm of scientific debate. Let him go to the secret chambers of his conscience for guidance, for his decisions are no longer an object of public concern, and the essence of belief is so much an inner and personal thing that no measure of general knowledge, of experience, of objective understanding, is applicable to it.

Natural science has no power over what is beyond the phenomenal world. It knows nothing of the origin of the world. Far back though it can reach with the aid of its data (and these reach back far beyond the beginnings of the human race), yet it has always as its object only the world as the Given, and its task is to fathom the history of the world within the confines of this Given. For a long time there has been general agreement that the natural history of the heavenly bodies should be based on mechanistic laws and on mathematical formulas, when at all possible. For a long time man has striven to discover similar laws for organic bodies and the world of the living, but for the most part in vain. Was it not justifiable to acknowledge special powers in these bodies, powers whose effects differed from the mechanistic behavior of the rest of nature? Man can make air and water, and fire and earth; should he not also be able artificially to make plants and animals, or even human beings, if they originate in a mechanistic fashion?

In vain did the learned man of medieval times strive to fabricate the homunculus. In vain our contemporaries seek for the means to make cells. The doctrine of spontaneous generation (*generatio equivoca*), according to which living beings are supposed to arise without father and mother from non-living material, is constantly losing ground, and only the lowest and most tiny of plant and animal organisms still offer a possibility of now renewing the old argument. For all of the most perfected organisms spontaneous generation has been discarded; every plant has its germ, every animal its egg or its bud, and every cell originates from an antecedent cell. It is just in recent years that we have succeeded in breaking the last supports of spontaneous generation in the natural history of disease, as we have learned to derive every new formation, every tumor, and every pathological growth from a parent structure proper to the healthy body.

Life thus forms a long, unbroken chain of generations, in which the child becomes the mother, and the effect becomes the cause. An interwoven chain of living parts within which an utterly complex, but nonetheless mechanistic, movement proceeds with constantly renewed youth and strength! Everywhere there is only propagation, nowhere a new beginning. The mechanistic movement of life is thus completely different from the chemical movement of the rest of nature, since in every case an already given organization, not artificially reproducible, forms the basis of the new organization issuing forth from it. To the extent that this movement continues under our eyes, it displays itself as something specifically differentiated and broken up into a great number of fixed lines among which no direct connection exists. The plant gives rise again to plants, the animal to animals. Furthermore, even the specific type of plant reproduces only plants of its own and of no other type; animals reproduce themselves only within their species. If the species dies out, it is extinct forever. Yes, even the disease product is bound up with the fixed and given limits of the type; even among the most deviant pathological circumstances, as I have tried to show, the human body generates no organic form and no cellular complex which does not have its counterpart in the healthy living process. All physiological and pathological formation is only the repetition, the now more simple, now more complex, reproduction of known, uniquely given patterns or types. *The plan of organization within the species is unalterable; type does not deviate from type.*

Hence, a new plan is not needed for every individual living creature about to be generated or born. The plan is already there in the maternal organism—bound to organic material—and the fact that it is realized, that it finally appears before our eyes in flesh and blood, is due to activity of material whose arousal is brought about in a completely mechanistic manner. Spiritualism cannot help us transcend this fact of experience.

But these types of living beings, these prototypes of the succeeding generations, were not always present. The history of our earth teaches us that type after type emerged into life; here, once again, the great difference between organic and inorganic nature shows itself. Nowhere do we find the beginning of the world, nor do we anywhere transcend the world. Life must have had a beginning, however, for geology leads us into epochs of the earth's formation in which life was impossible and neither trace nor sign of it is to be found. But if there was an origin of life, then it must be possible for science to fathom the conditions of this origin. At present this is an unsolved problem. Indeed, our experiences do not even justify us in regarding the invariability of species, which currently appears so certain, as a rule established for all time. For geology teaches us to recognize a certain hierarchial order in which species follow each other one after the other, higher after lower, and much as the experience of our time argues against it, I must still confess that it appears to me a scientific necessity to assume the possibility of a transition from species to species. Only then does the mechanistic theory of life achieve genuine security in this respect.

At present there is a great lack in our knowledge here. May we fill it out with speculations? Certainly, for only through speculation are investigative paths marked out in unknown fields. Admittedly, there is another way to fill out the gaps. One can take over the creation story from religious tradition, thereby simply trying to exclude investigation. But I say openly that no one has the right, even with the assumption of personal creation, to consider investigation into mechanistic processes inadmissible. That would be contrary to human nature and an attack on the mind. When even the positive religions picture the process of creation in a purely mechanistic manner, why do people wish to forbid science to comprehend these mechanics? If we cannot do otherwise than think mechanistically about natural processes, we ought not to be reproached when we apply this kind of thinking to the course of all natural events. That is the freedom of science, without which it would be fettered at every point of investigation.

But even in our own time a sufficient number of prophets of disaster can be found who foresee the greatest of dangers for State and Church arising from such an unleashing of Science. Is it still necessary to contradict them? When Science is untrue, does it not carry within itself the weapons to oppose falsehood? If the State as it is, and the Church as it has formed itself in the course of centuries, should not be able to stand the truth, would this not be a sure sign that they themselves have become untrue? Is it not Science which presses its way ever closer to knowledge of the truth, which preaches the rule of law more and more honestly? Truly, Science is dangerous only for the false, the arbitrary, the human ordinance. The more freely she yields herself to Nature, the greater the blessings she can pour out for mankind, and no epoch ought to be more committed to gratitude than precisely our own. It is not merely the material progress of peoples which she furthers. Superstition, the tendency to mysticism, and the prejudice of tradition are less and less in evidence. And in the place of mere negative enlightenment, always more surely, positive convictions of inner relatedness within the whole phenomenal world, of the steady progress of development, and of the solution of opposites in a higher unity, manifest themselves.

Atoms and Individuals

(1859)

PERMIT ME, HONORED GUESTS, to preface my treatment of the subject to which I wish to direct your indulgent attention with a few remarks not necessarily pertaining to it, but nevertheless perhaps not entirely without importance.

Like the human spirit, whose highest and most complete expression they are, languages have their peculiarities. They evolve with the development of the spirit; the more brilliantly consciousness unveils itself, the sharper become our expressions and the more transparent the meaning of our discourse. A language grows with a people; it reaches its highest perfection at the same time that the life of the people achieves its richest content and its supreme power. But the origin and formation of language is one thing, and its growth and development another. Language, indeed, resembles the spirit in this respect as well. The individual person can, in later years, cultivate the basic features of his spirit to a wonderful degree, but he cannot himself form new features. Similarly, the foundations of a language lie deep in the past history of a people; the greatest acumen of the scholar barely suffices to reach back to the earliest origin of the language-stems, and only with great effort is it possible to discover the roots from which, in a different manner for each family of peoples, the rich foliage of the tree of language has arisen. As it separates itself from its brothers, each people takes its inheritance of word-roots, or radicals, from the common treasury. These are its capital, and all further development of language is no more than a ceaseless derivation and combination, molding and transformation, adaptation and adornment, of something given once and for all. The

members of a people change; one generation replaces another and
the late arrivals forget the heritage into which they have entered.
Within the narrow or broadly drawn limits of a language, however, the spirit of a people reproduces itself faithfully as long as
this people remains true to itself. Language is the holiest treasure of a people, and shame be to those who wish to degrade it!

Many persons in Germany believe this at the present time;
we can hopefully say that more do with each succeeding day.
Therefore do not regard it as a desertion of the German spirit,
honored guests, if today I deliver a lecture whose title contains
nothing more than two foreign words. Permit me, rather, a few
additional remarks in order to present in general to this influential gathering a justification of science, which is so often berated
because of its preference for foreign words.

It is not because science is the property of all humanity, rather
than of a single people, that I justify this preference. This argument could avail only so long as science made general use of the
same language. Latin is dying out in science, however, just as the
people who spoke it have parted from us; the formal convention
of the learned, still sustaining the ancient tongue here and there,
continues to deteriorate with every upsurge of fresh popular life.
Everywhere science, too, returns to its native garments; the
strange cloak checks the free stride, and only in his mother tongue
is the scholar in a position to give freedom to the rapid flow of
thought. Only thus does his knowledge, adopting a national mode
of expression, overflow fully and fruitfully into the canals of
popular consciousness; the learned man, who once could find the
goal of his ambition only at the court of a prince, now stands
among an educated populace who give him not only honor but
assistance as well.

Neither prince nor people can give more than they have, however. And they do not have the new roots, the new radicals, required by the investigator for new discoveries and definitions in
the realms of mind and matter. They cannot tell him the names
of things neither seen nor thought of by anyone before his time.
Only the provincial dialects often maintain, with rare faithfulness,
the sharpest and most *characteristic* expressions for certain pecu-

liarities of life, but even these peculiarities have to be experienced or thought about. One thing more ought not to be forgotten. Language is not only an act of the spirit, but a fetter as well. As it at first favors the liberation of the spirit, so it later forms a tight net in whose fabric thought is ensnared. Only mathematics has succeeded in freeing itself; all other sciences are caught within. What is left for the investigator? When every kind of patching and alteration will no longer suffice, when the new conception cannot be introduced into the established speech-structure, there is no other way out except to borrow from another language. It certainly requires no explanation that science reaches back then, first of all, to those languages in which its earliest classic memorials were constructed, languages which both are no longer spoken and possess the greatest and most widely accessible store of roots. Here science can choose most freely, since attaching certain accessory meanings to the chosen word and fitting it out, so to speak, with an arbitrary content can be done independently. And at the same time there is the invaluable advantage of being able to select words that benefit to the same degree the educated speech of all peoples.

Thus many a Greek and Latin expression has been carried over into the speech of modern peoples by science, and has won the right of domicile. Every day we speak of atoms and individuals, for our language has no words that allow these things to be expressed with equal conciseness.

But just here we run into one of those peculiarities considered at the outset. Both words (atom and individual) in themselves mean precisely the same thing, yet they have entirely different connotations. Literally translated, the Greek word *atom* signifies something that can no longer be divided, that neither the hand nor the spirit is able to subdivide further anatomically. The Latin word *individual*, taken literally, also designates something that can no longer be divided. The Latin *individual* can indeed only be translated into Greek by the word *atom*, and Aristotle actually uses this word in the sense of *individual*. Both signify the indivisible, the one, the unity. But how many subsidiary ideas adhere to this unity!

Since the ancient days of Greek philosophy, *atom* in the narrower sense has designated the smallest and last unit of matter that would be reached if any given portion of a body were split up into smaller and smaller parts, although these last units can never really be reached because they lie beyond all possibility of sensual recognition. But atoms are not the ultimate parts of bodies in general; rather they are the ultimate parts of the elements from which these bodies are compounded. When the great—perhaps too great—number of chemical and physical elements of modern science was substituted for the four elements of antiquity, the conception of the atom changed in consequence. There are no atoms of fire or water today, but only atoms of ether, hydrogen, oxygen, and so forth, since these are the only substances whose elementary character we are able to recognize. The *monad* is unity in and for itself, but how much must be added to designate the particular monads called atoms! Modern science, in its poverty of language, has not forgotten even the monads, but it has treated them as it has the atoms; it has fitted them out with entirely new properties and peculiarities, and the philosophical monads of Leibniz are infinities away from the corporeal monads of Ehrenberg. While the monads of the philosopher are furthest to the left, or perhaps as one should say nowadays, furthest to the right, with respect to the ideal atoms of the physicist and the chemist, the monads of the scientific investigator align themselves beside individuals, sharing the old, well-founded rights.

What, then, are individuals? If it were only a matter of pointing out what is termed individual, this could quickly be done. But there are many kinds of things called individual, in both a good and a bad sense. Everybody speaks of individuals, of the individual person, of individuality. One refers to a human being, another to a plant; this one thinks about mind, that one about corporeal essence; many imagine individuality to be something great, others imagine it to be quite small; indeed, the question of whether atoms also are individuals has been seriously discussed. This confusion is present not only among the laity and the learned, among theologians and philosophers, among artists and critics, but even in the sanctum of natural science itself; it can be explained quite simply as the result of using the word not only in its true sense, but also in another sense, in which it is fitted out with a variety of accessory ideas. Although we want to pursue our topic here only from the standpoint of scientific investigation, nevertheless we must consider carefully all differences of opinion before seeking to establish a specific denotation. That we shall limit ourselves here to real things, following the general usage of language, will not be held against scientific investigators.

There is no doubt that individuals are not ultimate indivisible parts beyond the possibility of sensual recognition. On the contrary, we think here of visible, tangible bodies or beings often of such great spatial extent and of such complex structure that we can further distinguish in them systems, organs, and elements, the last of which can be subdivided still further, and whose smallest perceptible parts are in turn thought to be built up of innumerable atoms. In short, individuals are not ultimate particles but are unities with parts. Whence originates, then, their privilege of laying claim to indivisibility? What is the reason for ascribing individuality to them?

That the idea of the individual is to be sought for in the fact that, by its very nature, it may not be dismembered surely seems remarkable and points up a delicate subtlety of language. The atom is an indivisible unity that, even in thought, cannot be further divided; the individual is that which *may* not be further divided. If it is divided, it is at the same time destroyed. It is then no longer a unity in the individualistic sense, even though it still contains innumerable unities in the atomistic sense.

Therefore the parts of the individual, even the atoms, belong together; only in their togetherness, union, and community do they guarantee the total expression of individuality, only then do they fulfill that purpose which we are accustomed to associate with the total phenomenon.

The individual is, accordingly, a unified commonwealth in which all parts work together for a common end, or, as it might also be expressed, act according to a definite plan. As we have already pointed out, the parts themselves can be of very different character and significance, and our idea of the individual is so ambiguous that we can even take away parts of an individual thing without thereby eliminating our conception of it as such. Only certain decisive and important parts cannot be lacking. For us, a human being without arms or legs remains an individual; if he loses his head, thorax, or abdomen, however, we say: He was.

The atom is unchangeable and permanent; the individual is changeable and transitory. Atoms can enter into the most complicated combinations and groupings with other atoms, but they can withdraw again at any time with all of their properties intact. The individual depends on separation for its own maintenance; were it to submit itself fully to a union with another, it would necessarily surrender its individuality. Hence even its most intrinsic relationships retain a recognizable trace of exteriority; it can assimilate, to be sure, but it cannot allow itself to be assimilated. It has something that marks it off from its own kind as well as from other kinds, and which permits at the most an external union, however close. *Every individual, even though it belongs to a great group or array, has its particular characteristics.*

In what does this particularity consist? What is this "secret of individuality"? Before we attack this difficult question, let us consider for a moment, in order to make it more accessible, how far we may be permitted to extend the idea of the individual in the natural realm. Should we fill the whole of nature with individuality? Have the sun, the planets, the air and the sea, have stones and crystals, a claim to individuality? Many a modern philosopher and many a living scientist would answer Yes. Antiquity was universally of the same view, and even filled the whole of nature with its gods.

> Wo jetzt nur, wie uns're Weisen sagen.
> Seelenlos ein Feuerball sich dreht,
> Lenkte damals seinen gold'nen Wagen
> Helios in stiller Majestät.
> Diese Höhen füllten Oreaden,
> Eine Dryas lebt' in jenem Baum,
> Aus den Urnen lieblicher Najaden
> Sprang der Ströme Silberschaum.

But

Ach, von jenem lebenwarmen Bilde
Blieb der Schatten nur zurück.

.   .   .   .

Gleich dem todten Schlag der Penduluhr,
Dient sie knechtisch dem Gesetz der Schwere,
Die entgötterte Natur.[1]

Is it of any interest or value today to argue whether the sun
or the air are individual beings? They exist, and we rejoice in
them, but could they not be slightly different without any significant effect upon their separate existence? Would the sun not
remain the sun even if it had many more spots, or a much greater
circumference? Would the atmosphere cease to be the atmosphere
if it were full of carbon dioxide and nitrogen? Certainly this
would be very obvious to us, and perhaps the human race would
not survive, but this would be no basis for the lament that the
individual sun or the individual atmosphere had surrendered its
essence. For does not a soap bubble have as much right to individuality as a celestial body? Does it not obey the law of gravity
in just as servile a manner? Does not its entire existence depend
just as much on the universal necessity of attraction?

The individual is the converse of the general. Wresting itself
free from the necessity of universal law in order to find its own
law within, it strives after freedom and self-determination. Where
else, except in the organic world, is there freedom in nature? In
vain has an attempt been made to salvage individuality for crystals at least. Admittedly, external forces do not cause the parts
of crystals to order themselves together into beautiful forms;
external influences can affect the intrinsic forces pertaining to the
parts themselves, and can check, favor, or alter their activity.
Thus every crystal may have something particular and peculiar
in itself, but this particularity is not essential and does not reveal
its intrinsic character; it only indicates to us the external power
under whose pressure this intrinsic character has manifested itself,
and may even divert our attention from a consideration of the true
character of the crystal. But even where signs of external pressure
are least evident, and where the intrinsic forces generate the most

perfect of forms, is this form a necessary constituent of its true nature? Does the diamond not remain a diamond even though we cut it into a thousand artificially glittering surfaces under which its crystalline form gradually disappears? Is every one of its pieces not a diamond, no matter how many of them are struck out of the primary crystal? Is not a diamond only a particularly pure form in which carbon geologically appears, as the science of chemistry teaches us?

The individual is a living thing. Even the most magnificent crystal, though a paragon, is only a specimen. Without doubt, there are paragons among plants, animals, and even human beings, but they are such in a subsidiary sense, in the eyes of others. First and foremost they exist for themselves; everything that they become, they become from themselves, although not always through themselves. The peculiarity of "inwardness" determines their character. The outer form, directly derived from this, faithfully reveals this intrinsic character to us, if we are able to grasp and understand it. At the peak of its development the whole phenomenon of individuality carries within itself the stamp of unity. Multitudinous and complicated as the parts may be, all are parts of a real commonwealth in which each part is related to the other and requires the other, and does not win its full significance outside of the whole. As Aristotle said, life works toward a goal, and as Kant more precisely explained, this goal lies within—life itself is the goal. A crystal can grow to monstrous proportions if the conditions and material for its growth are present. But *Es ist dafür gesorgt, dass die Bäume nicht in den Himmel wachsen.*[2] The inner goal is simultaneously an external standard beyond which the development of living things does not go. Space and time have value and meaning only for living things, for only the living thing bears within itself the burden of self-preservation and self-development; only the living thing loses out when its intrinsic determinants fail to achieve a definite degree of development at a definite time. Thus the individual bears its goal and standard within; thus it reveals itself as a real unity in contrast to the merely conceptual unity of the atom.

However, it is not so easy for the investigator to grasp this unity. Let us not forget that the individual's unity rests on the commonwealth of its parts, and that this unity can be experienced, but cannot really be conceived without some insight into the manner of origin of those parts. Science makes syntheses, certainly, but only after it has analyzed; the first task of the investigator is to take things apart, to analyze, to anatomize; afterwards union, synthesis, and physiology follow. How long is the way and how many illusions it offers! We seek unity and find multiplicity; the organic structure disintegrates and crumbles in our hands, and in the end only the atoms remain. Is this really the right path to an understanding of the individual? Can we seek for a science of life where only death is to be found? Is this wholly disintegrative science of nature nothing other than a will-o'-the-wisp, and is it truly not high time that we turn aside to follow other paths?

If only there were others! But we have no choice! There is only one path of investigation, and it is the path of observation, dissection, and analysis, whether carried out on bodies or ideas. Admittedly, the scientific investigator can no more reassemble a plant or animal body that he has once taken apart than a boy can reconstruct a watch on which his youthful investigator's spirit has exercised itself. But nature is fruitful. Therefore let us go forward, for only from the parts can the Whole be understood!

The commonwealth of the individual is thus made up of a definite number—sometimes great, sometimes small—of necessary constituents. It is for this reason that we call it an organism. Concerning the organs, these necessary and active constituents, it has been known for a long time that they are ordinarily composed of smaller homogeneous (although not equivalent) parts. These have been called *similar parts*, and it can justifiably be said that the history of progress in our knowledge of the similar parts is simultaneously a history of the empirical doctrine of life, of physiology, and of biology in the broadest sense. It is a long story of laborious investigation in which one generation after another has worked with untiring zeal. With means at first very crude, then ever finer, an attempt has been made to understand the similar parts with respect to their form and structure, as well as their activity and effects, until at last, with the aid of the highly refined methods of physics and chemistry, we have succeeded in observing the most delicate manifestation of life. The similar parts of present-day biology are practically inaccessible to the naked eye; what the astronomer achieves in universal space with his telescope, this and even more the biologist achieves in the restricted space of the organism with the help of his microscope. The cells are his stars, and I hope that the time will come when the discovery of a new kind of cell will seem just as important as a new addition to the great number of tiny planets—perhaps even more important.

Two hundred years have already passed since cells were first recognized. A more precise knowledge of them, however, is scarcely two decades old; they are not yet established in science generally, and it is too much to ask that the new viewpoint should so soon be incorporated into the educated man's realm of ideas.

But it is precisely among us, to a greater extent than anywhere else, that this ought to be the case, for it is almost exclusively a merit of German science that the cell doctrine has become the basis of biology. Schleiden,[3] for the first time, undertook to trace plant life back to cells. Schwann,[4] at that time associated with our university, demonstrated the cellular composition and origin of the majority of animal tissues. Numerous investigators have followed them, and I have myself endeavored to solve the riddle of disease in terms of altered conditions of the cells, and to demonstrate the cellular unity of life in health and disease in both animals and plants. Everywhere that life is active, whether healthy or diseased, we meet with these tiny structures which present themselves in their simplest form as hollow vesicles possessing a delicate membrane distinguishable externally, a very complicated nucleus internally, with a highly variable content lying between.

All life is bound to cells, and the cell is not only the vessel of life but the living part itself. Indeed, every organic individual is replete with life. Life does not have its seat in this or that location; it does not reside only in one or another part. Not so—it is in all parts to the extent that they are of cellular origin. Not only are the nerves alive, not only is the blood, but even in flesh, bones, and hair there is vigorous life-activity, just as the root, the leaf, the flower, and the seed of the plant carry life within. How infinitely rich is this picture of life! At the Tiefenhof in Zürich stands an ancient linden tree; when it unfolds its crown of leaves every year it forms some ten trillion new living cells, according to the estimate of Nägeli. In the blood of an adult man, incidentally, sixty trillion extremely tiny cells circulate at every moment, according to the reckoning of Vierordt and Welcker. Full of humility, we gaze upward at the eternal stars to which even the earliest generations of mankind directed their prayers. But the wonders of nature are not only to be sought in this starry canopy; wonders greater and more difficult to explain continually take place within ourselves. Know thyself, mortal! Wrest from thyself the true humility of self-knowledge!

What is an organism? A society of living cells, a tiny well-ordered state, with all the accessories—high officials and underlings, servants and masters, the great and the small. In medieval times it was customary to say that an organism was a microcosm, a little world. Nothing of the sort! The cosmos is no replica of the human being, nor is the human being a replica of the world! Nothing resembles life except life itself. The state can be termed an organism, since it consists of living citizens; conversely the organism can be termed a state, or a family, since it consists of living members of like origin. But here the comparison is at an end. Nature is bifurcate; the organic is something quite special, something entirely different from the inorganic. Although built up from the same materials, from atoms of the same character, the organic world consists of an interconnected array of phenomena essentially split off from the inorganic world. Not that the latter represents "dead nature," since only something which once has lived can die. Inorganic nature too has its activity, a never-ending, brisk moving and shaping, endlessly effective and lively; but, except in a figurative sense, this activity is not life.

In comparison with the rest of nature, therefore, we feel ourselves to be something personal and set apart. But this sentiment is somewhat diminished by the realization that each one of us

represents a kind of society in himself, just as do plants and animals. Direct experience of the vigorous life which is active in all
of our parts is certainly most refreshing. Whoever has felt what
it means when a certain number of these cells, these involuntary
members of an organization, fail in their duty, whoever has had
his limbs crippled by some severe illness, knows well enough how
to value the pleasure felt when every member responds in its
turn with full and easy activity. But we desire still more; the
human heart is insatiable and the spirit strives against the desires
of the flesh. What, are we no more than an association of parts,
and is the organic individual without existence except as a commonwealth? Is this not contrary to our aesthetic judgment and
to our philosophical knowledge?

Indeed, the scientific investigator becomes involved at this
point in a very ticklish situation. Should he contradict the judgment of his senses? Should he turn aside from the path of investigation and with a sense of the inadequacy of all experience
bid farewell to experience? Let us remain calm! What is the
basis of the aesthetic judgment, and what is philosophical knowledge? The aesthetic judgment bases itself on the contemplation
of form; molding itself on the study of nature, it raises itself above
the bare aesthetic feeling by penetrating into the laws according
to which the forms are shaped. Therefore the aesthetic judgment
can never prescribe laws to natural science; it can only receive
them from or develop them together with science, and if it does
not do so, it is no more than prejudice resting on outmoded tradi-
tions, on hearsay and imposed doctrine. In aesthetics, too, true
judgment develops along with a better understanding of the laws
of form; although the profound feelings, the naïveté, and the
direct perception of the artist have not uncommonly preceded
scientific knowledge by thousands of years, we must nonetheless
recognize the distinction between the artist himself and the
art critic. True artists were never enemies of anatomical experience.

Even philosophical knowledge has no source for the understanding of nature other than scientific investigation. Inborn
knowledge does not exist, and the history of philosophy—of Ger-

man philosophy in particular—has satisfactorily demonstrated that an empty construction of nature from ideas is not feasible. Aristotle, Bacon, and Descartes were themselves investigators, or at least they comprehended the full range of the natural-scientific data of their periods. Our so-called nature-philosophy, in the narrower sense, has given birth only to confusion; it may be said of all our philosophers that their weakest writings are those in which they deal with the philosophy of nature. What reason have we therefore to be frightened by such misgivings?

These misgivings indeed are only small ones; for their contradiction it should suffice to point to the unequivocal testimony of men whose aesthetic and philosophical judgment is beyond question. "Every living thing," says Goethe, "is not single, but multiple; even in so far as it appears to us as an individual it remains nonetheless an association of living self-sufficient beings, which, though alike in idea or plan, can in their manifestations be identical or similar, unlike or dissimilar." Can one speak more clearly? And very acutely he continues: "The less developed the creature is, the more alike or similar are these parts and the more they resemble the whole. The more highly developed the creature becomes, the more dissimilar become the parts. The more alike the parts are, the less they are subordinated. Subordination of parts points to a more highly developed creature." He chooses the plant as an illustrative example: "That plants or trees," he says, "which appear to us as individuals, consist of numerous individual parts alike or similar to each other and to the whole— of this there is no doubt at all. How many plants are reproduced by shoots! The eye of the fruit tree brings forth a twig that produces in its turn a number of similar eyes; in precisely this same way reproduction through seeds takes place. It is the development of an innumerable host of similar individuals from the womb of the mother plant."

Hegel says of Goethe that his work on the metamorphosis of plants "formed the start of a rational consideration of the nature of plants, in that it shifted our attention from a preoccupation with mere fragments to a recognition of the unity of life." "The identity of organs," Hegel adds, "is predominant in the category

might say. After every autumn storm the sea throws up on our coast thousands upon thousands of jellyfish—peculiar masses of jelly whose rainbow colors surprise the eye. The females already carry living progeny originating from egg cells and able to swim about. If the animals remain in the depths of the ocean, the young ones take root after a time and grow into tiny polyps; saucer-shaped bodies form later on their free ends, one over another, developing more and more fully and at last breaking loose to swim about once again as jellyfish. Again and again the jellyfish produces eggs from which young polyps develop, and the polyps bring forth sprouts from which jellyfish arise.

But not all polyps multiply by budding. Some produce eggs and bring forth young in the usual manner. Many of them, moreover, may be artificially multiplied, like plants, with cuttings. Trembley[5] performed a celebrated experiment with the tiny fresh-water polyps of our ponds; he minced the creatures, and the bits again developed into polyps. But this is not all. In the Mediterranean there is a flourishing race of splendid, motile polyps, brought to the attention of the educated classes by Carl Vogt,[6] in particular. The young polyp develops from an egg. Swimming freely in the water, it begins to grow. To bear it up an air-filled bladder forms on its cranial end. On its caudal end an apparatus of feelers and tentacles, with curious stinging organs, develops in rich and beautiful profusion. In its continuously elongating trunk a longitudinal tube is to be found. Budlike sprouts arise from the trunk. Some of these form an array of swimming bells, moving themselves and thereby the whole creature. Others develop into new polyps, possessing mouths and stomachs; these not only gather nourishment for the whole organism, but also digest it, in order to surrender it at last to the common tube in the trunk. Finally, still other buds take on the appearance of jellyfish and attend to reproduction; they bring forth eggs from which free swimming polyps again arise. Where is the individual here? The young polyp appears primary to us, but from it grows a trunk like that of a plant. This trunk generates rootlike tentacles which move in a purposeful manner and seize prey; it forms a stalk with a nutritional canal, but no more than a plant does it have a mouth to make use of this canal. Like a plant it brings forth buds and sprouts, but each bud has particular tasks that are carried out with seemingly highly individualized activity. Special sprouts or branches, provided with their own motive power, attend to locomotion, others to the intake and digestion of food, and still others to reproduction. The trunk is nothing without its parts, and the parts nothing without the trunk. Which is the individual and which the organ? Are the organs individuals? Is the whole only a collection of individuals, a family, a colony, or even, as Vogt says, a phalanstery?

What a disorderly picture! What fragmentation of life! Everything that we are accustomed to think of in a single body, concealed as it were beneath a common exterior, lies here in open disconnection, exposed to the gaze of all. The whole individual is dispersed into a loosely held together mass of members, of individual bodies whose individual character is just as probable and again just as doubtful as that of the trunk, which has been entirely subordinated. Where is freedom here? Where is self-determination? Can we really accept these plant-animals as something to be compared with our closed, completely unified individuality? Should we measure our nature against such a lowly creature?

Permit me to answer with the words of the father of natural science: "We must proceed," says the teacher of Alexander the Great, "with the investigation of every kind of animal without wrinkling up our noses, since there is something natural and admirable in everything. For existence itself—determined not by blind chance but by the idea of purpose—is to be found in the works of Nature alone, but the goal for which things exist, or have come into being, dwells primarily in the realm of the beautiful. Should anyone hold that the study of other animals is a low thing, then he must also hold the same opinion with respect to himself, for it is not possible to look at the parts which compose the human being—the blood, flesh, bones, vessels, and similar parts—without great repugnance. But one must bear in mind that whoever works with any of the parts or vessels does not conceive of his investigation as stopping with the study of this material; he is not concerned with it alone, but rather with the whole form—just as one might think in terms of a house, rather than bricks, mortar, and wood, so the natural scientist must be concerned more with the structure and the whole nature of the thing than with something never found dissociated from it. First of all, it is necessary to ascertain within every species those phenomena that, as such, apply to all animals; only then may one attempt to delve into causes."

Let us move upward one step, from the invertebrates to the vertebrates. Here, as everywhere else in the whole scale from the lowest fish up to the human being, there is a common plan of organization. No clusters of plants or plant-animals, only self-contained individuals! The higher we climb in the class of vertebrates, the more definitely the unified phenomenon of the individual confronts us, until at last it achieves its subjective conclusion, and therewith convincing certainty, in the human consciousness. The scientific investigator is not impervious to subjective experience, but he recognizes as certain only those inner experiences in whose comprehension the subject treats itself, in the true philosophical sense, as an object of impartial observation. Now, from this standpoint, what can we allow?

To the scientific investigator, just as to the philosopher or anyone else, consciousness is a fact which is as certain as it is inexplicable. To designate it a property of the soul explains just as little as to insist that it is a property of the brain, or to say of weight that it is a property common to all bodies. To determine the nature of weight, it is not enough to demonstrate that it manifests itself in a universal mutual attraction of all massy particles; rather, we must show what leads the massy particles to attract each other. Although we are in no position to point this out, nevertheless we rightfully use gravity as a basis for the explanation of many processes in the heavens and on the earth, and we can do likewise with consciousness. Here, however, a considerable barrier stands in our way. Weight is an attribute of all bodies; consciousness is neither an attribute of all individuals (since plants, and a large number of animals, certainly do not offer us the slightest justification for ascribing consciousness to them), nor a constant attribute of human beings, since often enough we observe

states of unconsciousness; finally, consciousness is not an attribute
of the whole man, for experience shows us that it is closely bound
to the brain. Still worse, even in its most fully developed state,
consciousness is limited to a relatively small fraction of the processes actually occurring in the body. If we had not gradually succeeded, in the course of objective research pursued for millennia,
in making even the most hidden states of our own bodies accessible
to observation, the content of our consciousness would be extremely meager. When, as the result of injury, a human being
has the misfortune to suffer an interruption of continuity in his
spinal marrow, his consciousness of all processes taking place in
parts of his body whose nerves enter the spinal marrow below
the point of injury immediately ceases; every influence of the will
is extinguished here, yet these parts live and the individual persists.

*Consciousness of self, therefore, is only the subjective—not
the objective—unity of the individual.* This consciousness is not
the mover but the moved. It is not the effective power in the
body, the power that actualizes the plan of organization and the
purpose of the individual; on the contrary, it appears to be the last
and highest product of life, the finest fruit of the long chain of
interconnected processes determining the history of the individual. The individual as a corporeal being, in the fullness and
luxuriousness of its life, must of necessity be inwardly composite;
only in this way are development (the progress from lower to
higher states) and perpetuation of new forms of life assured.
Life must be the collective product of the activity of all its individual parts, and all of these parts must in themselves have something general as well as something special. Without the general
features which must prove to be equally characteristic of every animal and plant, the idea of life would cease to be equally applicable
to all; without special features, life would be everywhere the
same. *The human individual is also a commonwealth.*

Scientific investigation reveals the individual to be composed
of an array of systems; one attends to sensations, another to movements, others to the intake of nourishment and air, some support
the parts and others bind them together, and so on. Every one

of these systems comprises a certain number of special organs; every organ includes a number—usually limited—of tissues, and every tissue is in the end composed of cell regions and cells. The "I" of the philosopher is a consequence of the "We" of the biologist. It would lead me too far afield at this point if I attempted to enumerate all of the reasons leading to the conclusion that, in the human body as elsewhere, cells and their derivatives are the truly active parts, that life dwells in each one of these, that each one possesses a certain degree of self-sufficiency, and that all living phenomena rest on the activity, on the cooperation or opposition, on the inactivity or destruction, of certain additive cellular unities. *Without doubt, the secret of individuality consists in the fine differences of plan and development of single cells or cell groups.* As in the lives of nations, so in the lives of individuals the state of health of the whole is determined by the well-being and close interrelation of the individual parts; disease appears when individual members begin to sink into a state of inactivity disadvantageous to the commonwealth, or to lead parasitic existences at the expense of the whole. Disease destroys all illusions about the substantial unity of the organism; illness and recovery are only possible as long as life remains intact in a certain residiuum of active healthy parts in the larger commonwealth.

Now are the cells or the human beings individuals? Can a single answer be given to this question? I say No! But I ask that this not be understood to mean that scientific investigation is in no position to offer a definite explanation. The difficulty is rather that the word *individual* came into use long before we possessed clear conceptions of the beings grouped together under this heading. The conception is therefore not sharply defined, and everyone is at liberty to interpret it in a narrow or broad sense, according to the degree of sensitivity with which his experience has disclosed to him the phenomena of individual existence. The conception of the *atom* as the ultimately conceivable particle is certain and unalterable, but it is not derived from direct experience like the conception of the *individual*, which has become vague and ambiguous with the broadening of that experience. If a decision to distinguish between collective individuals and single individuals (which would be the simplest way out) cannot be agreed on, then either the conception of the *individual* in the organic branches of natural science must be given up or it must be strictly bound to the cell. Systematic materialists, as well as spiritualists, if they are consequent in their logic, must arrive at the former conclusion, while it seems to me that an unprejudiced, realistic view of nature leads to the latter, since only in this way is a unified conception of life secured throughout the whole realm of plant and animal organisms. And precisely this appears to me as the first and most important requirement of all nature study, for it is the point at which the realistic efforts of the simple investigator link up with the idealistic wishes of the thinker who desires to set forth the plan of creation with the help of natural history. Present-day scientific investigation, like a grand jury, sits in judgment over the facts; it judges them, however, not as individual events but as members of an orderly interconnected series.

The consideration of organic creation leads us back, from generation to generation, in the long line of descent of the living, far beyond the darkness of the oldest chronicles, far beyond the beginning of the human race, into the stony past of the earth. We see the feeble beginnings of the plant kingdom, we find traces of animal types long since extinct, and later, much later, we encounter the lord of creation. According to geology, millennia adding up to millions of years passed by before individual cells developed into those greater commonwealths in which instinct and finally consciousness broke through. The recorded history of knowledge shows us how marvelously rich the positive contents of consciousness became in the course of a few thousand years. Though the histories of peoples and states in their rise and fall fill our spirit with pain and doubt, though with trepidation we ask ourselves daily whether affairs are improving or are they rather deteriorating, whether the human race is not hurrying toward its downfall and culture toward its own extinction, nevertheless true science shows only progress. States perish and peoples disappear under the boot of the conqueror; science remains to drive forth new and hardier shoots among those who but yesterday were barbarians. Annually the leaves of trees wither away in order that new and more highly developed blossoms may be produced in the following year; daily the blood cells in the human body are changed so that fresh elements may begin anew the work of their own dissolution. In like manner peoples wither and the children of mankind change; the following generation understands itself and nature better, consciousness becomes more secure, the *individual* becomes more free and powerful, ever more completely controlling the *atom*! With the realization that intellectual development is also an inseparable part of life, the human being regains that respect for his bodily existence which a gloomy world view, turned away from light and life, only too easily endangers. He who knows that the highest goal of life can only be reached when innumerable discrete parts, provided with the quality of individual existence and passing from generation to generation with continual renewal, work together toward a common goal, finds within himself the much sought for yet unexpected harmony that is satisfying at once to the understanding and the emotions, and is as much a standard for, as an instigation to, ethical action.

Standpoints in
Scientific Medicine

(1877)

IT WAS JUST THIRTY YEARS AGO, in April 1847, that under this same title I wrote the first paper for the initial issue of these Archives. Now, as we begin the 70th volume, if I recall a time lying so far in the past, I do so with the wish that the younger generation now beginning to contribute to the progress of science may look back with us at the goals which their elders set up a generation ago and have since unwaveringly pursued.

At that time we attempted to shake off the spell which philosophy, nature-philosophy in particular, had for a long period cast over science. We fought against *a priori* speculation; we rejected systems, and we relied solely on experience. It was not long before we were reproached for contributing to the decline of science, for putting an endless array of bare and detailed facts in the place of ordered knowledge, and for ruthlessly sacrificing millennia of practice on the altar of natural science without offering the helpless beginner a firm basis for his actions.

We did not permit ourselves to be frightened by either the number or the stature of our opponents. Undisturbed, we confined ourselves to the investigation of isolated problems, completely confident that every new fact would necessarily spread light in fields as yet dark, and that every forward step would to some extent increase our insight into the sequence of natural events and thereby broaden our view of natural processes. And we were not deceived. The medicine of today so little resembles the medicine of that time, and differs so greatly from two thousand years of traditional medicine, that it is already considered an indication of special erudition today when someone still commands a full and unprejudiced understanding of the past. How few among physicians of the present day are able to place themselves in the spirit of an era which did not yet know that capillaries are real vessels with definite walls, that organic muscle fibers are the bearers of movement even in the smallest organoid formations of the body, and that the delicacy of the peripheral nerve network exceeds even the boldest speculations! Yes, how few suspect that the period when all of this was unknown lies only thirty years behind us! What an effort it has cost to overturn a system of humoral pathology secured by a thousand bonds of language and popular tradition, and to set up in its place a straightforward science based on direct experience with a realistic view of the tissues and their significance for pathology and therapy! What efforts had to be made, what ever-renewed and minute investigations, in order to introduce the genetic principle into pathology, to establish the developmental history of individual processes, and to assign every phenomenon, whether it belonged to the progressive or regressive, the active or passive, the nutritive, formative, or functional category, to its proper place! And yet we have succeeded in bringing firm order out of seeming chaos; the thousands of individual facts have been comprehended in a few well-established laws and made easily accessible to the understanding of the younger generation in this new order.

True, we were enemies of tradition, but we have been justified with the passage of time. We were not, however, such barbarians as to consider it proper, as many do today, to despise or even ignore tradition merely because it is tradition. On the contrary, we were convinced that the only genuine knowledge is historical knowledge, that justice toward others is the only counterweight for exaggerated self-esteem, and that valuable lessons can be drawn from the study of error. We have not forgotten these things. As different from tradition as what we worked out was, yet we were proud to establish its connection with the verified part of the old science, and to seek out the sources lying behind us from which the newer point of view had taken origin.

He who has only once through his own efforts tried to trace back the long path trod by his predecessors, who has felt how clear and luminous his own knowledge becomes as he grows aware of the historical circumstances out of which it has arisen, and who discovers the basis of the errors by which even genuine investigators have been misled, he who has learned that a kernel of truth sticks in every error, will not place himself with those who despise historical studies. Admittedly, however, history which is satisfied by the parading forth of an array of fragmented and disconnected groups of statements from all periods in order to appear erudite, history without that genuine insight into the significance of what has been said, which can be understood only in the light of its time and in terms of the scientific presuppositions then considered valid, amounts to nothing. We older ones know well enough from our own painful experience how to appreciate this difference, since we are only too well able to evaluate the sort of nonsense that can be ascribed to a man of an earlier era when someone extracts a few scattered statements and trys out his newly acquired wisdom on them.

We were enemies of philosophy, to be sure, but not of philosophy in general, only of the cocksure, all-knowing, self-satisfied philosophy of the forties. We did not find our method—the currently accepted scientific method—without philosophy. We had respect not only for the "logic of facts," but for logic in general; we exerted ourselves to take up the old well-founded and thoroughly worked out logic, rather than to adjust our standard to the demands of a self-developed logic new for each special case. We were not blind to the advantages of dialectic. We sought for clear-cut conceptions, precision of expression, and correct terminology. We exerted ourselves to introduce a scientific language into medicine and to put our newly won understanding beyond the reach of wanton distortion, whether by impressions of the moment, by improper generalization, or by the tendency to the figurative misuse of conceptions.

Today it seems at times as if these were foolish concerns, since no one any longer pursues logic and dialectic. Should someone still have an inclination in this direction, he is offered "medical logic" instead of general logic. Ever and again terminology becomes confused. Hardly had success been achieved in clearly outlining the history of fatty metamorphosis and caseous transformation, after a long effort, when fatty degeneration and caseation were exaggerated, intermingled, and brewed into a mixture in which no one is any longer able to distinguish the elements. For many years we strove to bring about the recognition of white blood cells, lymph corpuscles, and lymph gland cells by defining the characteristics and pointing out the differences of each. At that time few were inclined to follow us on this path, but nowadays every round cell is a white blood cell and every white blood cell a lymph corpuscle; beyond this hardly anything special remains.

It is the same blind mania of imitation and schematization which has appeared, in a most terrifying fashion, in the "foundations" of men of finance in recent years. Where one factory for railway supplies flourished, ten more had immediately to be set up without anyone's considering that the same need does not require a tenfold satisfaction. Because one or the other contagious illness is caused by bacteria, immediately all contagion is bacterial.

In this connection nothing has had a more devastating effect than the crude schematization of the Darwinists. It was certainly somewhat surprising, for those of us who were still acquainted with the old nature-philosophy, to see how the genius of a single man restored to its rightful place an idea already given official status as an *a priori* necessity by the nature-philosophers, not only reactivating it, after its long and alas not entirely unjustified banishment, but making it the basis of a general conception of the history of the organic world. But to make an article of faith out of a problem, a principle of synthesis out of a ground for investigation, thereby drugging oneself with assumptions instead of seeking further, was almost worse than the *a priori* approach of the nature-philosophers. For all the valid facts which had been brought out in the meantime were also forced into the new system, and in this context they ran a very definite risk of losing their true meaning under a cloak of hypothesis. To many people the "struggle for existence" seemed to be something entirely new and unheard of, just as if the doctrine of self-preservation and the instinct of self-preservation had not always been the basis of biology. Even the doctrine of heredity, a phenomenon so commonplace in pathological experience, in its new form dazzled many an otherwise poorly illumined eye. The attempt to consider pathological heredity from an entirely new standpoint led many young workers in our science into displays of erudition which, singularly enough, were submitted least often to the journals of pathology.

May I recall in this connection that I belong to those who did not require this new stimulus in order to conceive of the variability of species as a necessary presupposition of the mechanistic theory of life? In a lecture on the mechanistic conception of life, which I gave at the 1858 Congress of Natural Sciences in Karlsruhe, one year before the appearance of the first edition of the *Origin of Species*, I expressed this view in the most clear-cut manner. In fact, as early as 1849 I had emphasized as a logical necessity the mechanical origin of all life out of general movement. Thus I have always been ready and willing to accept in a friendly manner and to treasure as a valuable acquisition every fact which illustrates the variability of the species and the primal creation. But I cannot avoid voicing a forceful warning, based on my own experience, against taking hypotheses for facts and forgetting the necessity for factual proof of particular cases because of the ease of general explanations.

Nothing was simpler, nothing more logical, nothing more closely in correspondence with the generality of natural-scientific views, than the doctrine of the origin of tissue components from chemical substances, from the so-called blastemas or histogenetic materials. When the Archives started, the descriptions of Schleiden concerning the origin of plant tissue elements, and those of Schwann concerning the origin of animal elements, had just attained general currency. The new "cell theory" was the old doctrine of *generatio equivoca* or epigenesis applied to formative processes within the plant and animal organism. The field for this cell theory was nowhere more favorable than in pathology. Every day brought a new confirmation of this theory in the form of seemingly quite factual observations concerning the organization of exudates and the primitive blastema. Appearances were so convincing that one could only wonder why all of this had not been recognized long before. And yet all of this has been proved false. From all of those investigations, carried out with the greatest devotion and care, absolutely nothing valid remains as regards the earliest origins of pathological new formations.

Nothing is more instructive in this connection than a scrutiny of the publications of my too soon departed friend Reinhardt,[1] in particular those concerning the genesis of the microscopic components of inflammatory formations and the so-called splitting of cell nuclei. One must have been, as I was, eyewitness to the tireless observational activity, throughout night and day, of this strict and conscientious man in order to experience with me in full the feeling of regret that so much work was carried out in vain, and indeed only because a theory in itself plausible, and perhaps in certain instances and with certain modifications applicable, had misdirected the observer's attention from the beginning. Questions based on false premises doom even the best pieces of work. A deficiency in logic is not always responsible for the false preises, although this is the case often enough. Much more often the inclination, inherent in mankind, to overhasty generalizations of views correct in themselves directs the observation away from the unprejudiced perception of events and makes the investigator biased.

What I said about Reinhardt also applies to Schwann himself. The imperishable laurels of these men were not won in the fields where their names resounded with the greatest acclaim from their contemporaries. It was not in the developmental history of pathological formations but in the sequence of retrogressive changes that Reinhardt was responsible for definitive and permanent progress. His paper concerning the origin of granular cells, in the first volume of the Archives, should be read carefully at least once by every physician interested in the historical development of knowledge. And what makes Schwann immortal is not the "cell theory," not the doctrine of the origin of "hourglass forms" from the "cytoblastema," but the demonstration of the cellular origin of all tissues. Later we were able to build on this demonstration, when, as a result of daily observation, the heretical thought of the continual reproduction of cells within the organism gradually germinated and grew. These thoughts became the basis of cellular pathology. But I myself needed five more years before I made the first hesitant attempts to proclaim them publicly. Only in the third issue of the fourth volume of the Archives[2] did I begin to break the spell of the "cell theory," and only in the eighth volume did I achieve a presentation of the new standpoint with some degree of freedom.

Such reminiscences are well suited to call forth in the younger generation a certain degree of caution—even more, of conservatism. May they at least help to explain my own conservatism with respect to newer theories! Many have asked me in surprise why I am not a Darwinist, since my own ideas touch on those of Mr. Darwin. I can only reply that I am a Darwinist at heart just as I am a cosmopolitan at heart. However, just as this inner cosmopolitanism, or, let us say, humanism, does not prevent me from harboring good national sentiments and from feeling in many ways first of all a German, so in science I am first of all a pathologist, and as such I must strongly emphasize that *pathological formations never develop beyond the physiological possibilities of the species.* In pathology there is no such thing as heterology in the Darwinian sense. The heterology of development (heteroplasia) which I defend, and as whose foremost proponent I may be permitted to regard myself, applies only to the tissues and not to the species. All the facts we know allow us to recognize a histological, but not a geneological, change in pathology. And therefore I claim that just as the doctrine of *generatio equivoca* is no longer applicable to histopathology since the disappearance of the "blastema," so the doctrine of the variability of species is impermissible in pathology since the eclipse of the so-called "cell theory." In no way does this imply, however, that outside of histopathology and pathology in general, epigenesis or transmutation of the species may not occur.

What we should have grasped in the course of the past generation is, above all, that pathology must be an independent science. The elaboration of the idea that it would not suffice to conceive of pathology as applied physiology, and that we needed rather a pathological physiology with its proper field of work and independent activity, forms a not inconsiderable part of the leading article with which the Archives were inaugurated thirty years ago. My considerations were directed essentially against the so-called "rational" medicine and the self-designated "physiological" school, movements at that time in full flower. It was an unpleasant task to turn away from paths pursued by talented and industrious men. Now that the task is finished, we should also bear in mind that the emancipation of pathology, and its elevation to the rank of a natural science, requires above all else that pathologists guard their independence and let no foreign science arbitrarily intrude its hypotheses into pathology, if pathology is not to be relegated again to the position of a mere applied science. We can do this *only if we remain at our tasks and accomplish something*. As always, there will be no better sign that we are working productively than the delivery of useful fruits to related scientific disciplines, above all to anatomy and physiology. We must be able to give them of our riches; we cannot permit ourselves to sink back again to the state of desiring nothing more than a share in the wealth of others.

It is no longer necessary today to write that scientific medicine is also the best foundation for medical practice. It is sufficient to point out how completely even the external character of medical practice has changed in the last thirty years. Scientific methods have been introduced everywhere into practice. The diagnosis and prognosis of the physician are based on the experience of the pathological anatomist and the physiologist. Therapeutic doctrine has become biological and thereby experimental science. Concepts of healing processes are no longer separated from those of physiological regulatory processes. Even surgical practice has been altered to its foundations, not by the empiricism of war, but in a much more radical manner by means of a completely theoretically constructed therapy.

And thus we can welcome with happy hearts the little anniversary which the Archives now celebrates, as it places itself at the disposal of a second generation. May coming generations seek their honor in equaling the one which now retires! The Archives will in the future reckon it a particular honor to introduce not only new schools of thought, but also new individual voices, to the scientific world. All of them require outside help for their first steps. Many a new school of thought which first gained strength and recognition in these Archives has afterwards created its own journal; many an investigator whose useful works appeared in the Archives has later started his own publication. Let there be a friendly greeting to all! For even the strong can maintain their strength undiminished only with competition and constant exercise.

The Place of Pathology
Among the Biological Sciences

(1893)

IT IS NOW ALMOST TEN YEARS since this illustrious society[1] conferred on me the unexpected honor of election to foreign member-
ship. Not only this, but last autumn it considered me worthy of
an additional honor when it awarded me the Copley medal—a
sign of the highest recognition, the significance of which far exceeds those distinctions which the changing favor of political
power is accustomed to bestow. Nevertheless, deeply as I appre-
ciated this mark of its constant and ever-increasing esteem, I was
still not in a position to offer my thanks in person to the society.
Numerous duties, official as well as private, the burden of which
has increased each year, have kept me continuously working at
home, and even during vacation the freedom of my movements
has been for some time restricted by international engagements
which become more numerous and pressing each year.

With great indulgence, which I very much appreciate, your
executive committee has allowed me to postpone the date of my
appearance before you. Hence you see me among you today, for
the first time, to tell you in person how grateful I am to the society, and how great an incentive to new efforts your recognition
has been.

Who among us does not need friendly encouragement in the
changing circumstances of life? Genuine happiness, it is true, is
not based on the appreciation of others, but rather on one's own

consciousness of honest labor. How otherwise could we stand fast in the midst of the daily turmoil? How could we retain the hope of progress and final victory in the face of the attacks of our opponents and in the face of the insults spared to no one who appears in public life? He who is exposed to public opinion during a long and busy life surely learns to bear unjust criticism with equanimity, but this rests only on the confidence that his cause is just and must some day triumph. This is our hope in our struggle for progress in science and art; this is our hope in our battle for civil and religious liberty, and with this hope we gradually become hardened against malicious attacks. It is a kind of immunization which, I admit, has great disadvantages, for insensitivity to unjust attacks very easily leads to a similar indifference to just attacks, and even, in keeping with the perverse tendency rooted in the nature of human thought, finally leads to indifference alike to praise and recognition. We withdraw taciturnly into ourselves, discontented both with the world and with ourselves, for who can so completely retire within himself that a realization of the insufficiency of human thought and of the legitimacy of hostile criticisms cannot penetrate the crust of his consciousness, however hard it may become? Happy is he who has strength enough to preserve or regain his relations with other men, and to take part in the common work! Thrice happy he who does not lack in this work the commendation of highly respected colleagues!

Such were the thoughts which filled my mind as I reviewed my own life and the history of our science in anticipation of the present occasion—or, to put it otherwise, as I surveyed the fortunes of our predecessors. How often have I found myself in a despondent state, beset by a feeling of extreme depression! And the history of our science—what long periods of stagnation and what numerous interruptions due to the victory of erroneous doctrines it has endured! What saved me was the habit of work, a habit which did not forsake me even in times of external misfortune, the habit of scientific work which has always appeared to me as a recreation after tiring and fruitless efforts in political, social, and religious fields.

What has saved science is the same thing; it only seems different because the cooperation of many is necessary to make progress secure; hence the exalting and consoling thought that one nation after another appears on the scene to share in the task. When the star of science becomes dim in one country, sooner or later it shines so much the brighter elsewhere. Thus one nation after another becomes the teacher of the world.

No science has gone through these waxings and wanings of brilliancy more often than medicine. It is the only one of the sciences which, in the course of a development lasting for more than 2,000 years, a development often disturbed yet never completely arrested, has always found a new home. To illustrate this with examples drawn from the whole of the past would lead us too far afield. For my present purpose it suffices to make the chief features of modern medicine the object of our attention. Cursory as it must be, such a sketch should at the same time throw some light on the intellectual relations of our two nations, the English and the German, for both have taken a prominent part in establishing the fundamental principles of modern medicine.

The downfall of the old medicine, the so-called humoral pathology, was brought about in the beginning of the sixteenth century. In Germany we are inclined to attribute to our country a decisive role in this memorable struggle. It was a man of our race, Andreas Vesalius ("der Weseler"), who made anatomy an exact science, and thus with one stroke gave medicine a solid foundation, on which it has since remained and which it will, let us hope, never lose.

But the main blow at ancient medicine was struck by his somewhat elder contemporary Paracelsus—at once a charlatan and a gifted physician who erased from the beliefs of mankind the doctrine of the four humors which, pseudo-chemical in its construction, was the foundation of the old pathology. He accomplished this, curiously enough, with weapons borrowed from the arsenal of the Arabs, the successors of the Greek physicians and the chief representatives of medieval humoral pathology. He borrowed alchemy from them also, and at the same time the fantastic spiritualism of the East, which found its most distinct expression in the doctrine of the *archaeus* as the determining force in all living beings. Thus the new medicine, at its very birth, took up the seeds of that ruinous antagonism leading to the embittered strife of the schools which persists into our own century.

To Vesalius we owe that spirit of exact inquiry beginning from the observation of actual conditions, which, without further ado, we may designate "anatomical." Paracelsus, who called the anatomy of the dead body useless, and who sought for the basis of life as the highest goal of knowledge, demanded "contemplation" before everything else. Just as he himself arrived by this path at the metaphysical construction of the *archaei*, so he loosed among his followers a wild and completely fruitless mysticism.

Nevertheless, hidden in his "contemplation" lay a healthy kernel, which did not allow the intellectual activity aroused by it to sink back to rest. This was the idea of *life*, which formed the ultimate problem of all future research. Curiously enough, this idea, which has always persisted in the popular imagination and is to be found in an unmistakable form even among primitive nations, had been forced far into the background in scholastic medicine. Since the time of Hippocrates, it had been the custom to use, instead of "life," the obscure expression φύσις, *natura*; but it is useless to seek for an exact definition of this term. To Paracelsus nature was alive, and the basis of this life was that very *archaeus*, a force different from matter and separable from it, a spirit (*spiritus*), as he himself expressed it, in accordance with the Arabs. In the complex human organism, the "microcosm," each part, in his opinion, had its own *archaeus* and the whole was governed by the *archaeus maximus*, the *spiritus rector*. On this basis originated that long succession of vitalistic schools, which, in everchanging forms, and with constantly new terminology, have introduced into the minds of physicians the notion of a basic lifeprinciple.

If the sagacious Georg Ernst Stahl,[2] whose services to the development of chemistry are now universally acknowledged, substituted the soul for the *spiritus rector*, and so created a system of animism, the last vestiges of which have only in our own time disappeared from the school of Montpellier, so did the pure vitalists in turn build up on the basis of the dogma of specific

dynamic forces, maintained so stoutly by the physicists, that notion
of the life-force, whose half-spiritualistic and half-physical character contributed so much, even up to our own time, to the
confusion and puzzlement of men's minds. The doctrine of the
life-force found its strongest support in nature-philosophy, especially in that variety which soon obtained general sovereignty in
Germany.

This summary exposition has greatly anticipated the historical
course of the development of medicine. It is now appropriate to
pay proper homage to that great investigator who made the exact
method the rule, and at the same time to acknowledge the importance of the country which gave him birth in determining the
new direction of our science. Nearly one hundred years had
passed since Vesalius and Paracelsus had done their work when
William Harvey published his *Exercitatio Anatomica de Motu
Cordis et Sanguinis in Animalibus.* Here, for the first time, the
anatomical examination of living parts was carried out, in masterful style and according to the experimental method. All objections
that anatomy concerned itself only with dead parts were set aside
with one stroke; living activity became the object of direct observation. This was carried out on one of the most important
organs, one absolutely necessary for life, one whose varying activity constantly attracts the attention of the general practitioner.
Not only this, but also a new method of observation—the experimental method—was introduced into research, a method with
which a new branch of medical science, physiology, has been
laboriously built up.

The influence of this marvelous discovery of Harvey's on the
ideas of his contemporaries and successors was very great. Among
his contemporaries the last support of Galenism fell with the
demonstration of the circulation; among his followers an understanding of the course of local processes began to dawn. Ancient
and extremely difficult problems, such as that of inflammation,
could now be attacked anew. A goodly part of life became intelligible, since a living organ itself had now been subjected to observation, and, to the astonishment of all, its activity turned out
to be completely mechanical. The revolution of thought was so

far-reaching that it has since become almost impossible even to picture the ideas of the older physicians to whom the circulation of the blood was unknown.

Nevertheless, in spite of such striking results, the desire for a more complete understanding remained unsatisfied. The action of the living heart could be observed—but how did it live? What was this life, whose activity one observed? In the heart itself, the essence of life could not be found.

Harvey directed his attention to another subject; he tried to observe the first beginnings of life in hatched eggs of birds and in mammalian embryos. In this way he soon came to the question of the general significance of the ovum, and enunciated the celebrated dictum, "Omne vivum ex ovo." In the light of the more extensive research of modern investigators this dictum has turned out to be too restricted for the whole animal kingdom, and imprecise in its application to plant life. But its validity with respect to the higher animals cannot be questioned, and it has become one of the firm points on which investigation of sexual differences and reproduction has been based. Because of the imperfections of his optical instruments, Harvey was unfortunately not able to see what he was really trying to investigate, namely, the process of organization as such, just as he had previously been unable to recognize the continuity of the capillary circulation. These imperfections were to persist for a long time, and thus it came about that even Albrecht von Haller and John Hunter[3] considered the formation of the area vasculosa in the hatched eggs of birds to be the beginning of organization, and even as the type of organization itself.

I must return to this point later; for the moment I should like first to direct your attention to a man whose importance for the further development of the doctrine of life has always seemed to me to have been particularly great and significant, but who has, nevertheless, sunk into unmerited oblivion—not only among posterity in general, but also, I think I may say, even in the minds of the majority of his countrymen. I refer to Francis Glisson,[4] Harvey's contemporary, whose works appeared almost at the same time as those of his celebrated colleague; but the brilliancy

of Harvey's discoveries was so great that the light shining from
Glisson's work-table was almost eclipsed in comparison. I rejoice
that on so auspicious an occasion I can recall the memory of this
modest investigator, and pay the debt of gratitude which science
owes him.

Thirty-five years ago, when I published my little essay "Irritation and Irritability,"[5] I knew little more of Glisson that what
every medical student learns, namely, that the liver has a "capsula
communis Glissonii," and, what is less well known, that he had
written a small work on rickets, the first of its kind. In my own
paper on this disease[6] I pointed to the care and accuracy which
characterize his book and make it a model for the summarizing
of investigative data, but even then I overlooked the fact that this
was only the least merit of this extraordinary man. Only in the
course of further studies on the history of the doctrine of irritation and irritability did I make the discovery, most surprising to
me, that the notion of irritability did not stem from Haller, as is
generally believed, but that the father of modern physiology, and
the Leyden school from which he came, had borrowed this conception from Glisson. I then stumbled on a series of almost
forgotten publications of this original scholar, in particular his
*Tractatus de natura substantiae energeticae, seu de vita naturae
ejusque tribus primis facultatibus, perceptiva, appetitiva et motiva*[7] (London, 1672) wherein ideas whose main features had
already been presented in his *Anatomia Hepatis* (1654) were
elaborated. In this work the newly coined word *irritabilitas* appears in the literature for the first time, as far as I know. It may
be mentioned, in this connection, that the expression *irritatio* is
much older. I find it as early as Celsus, but with an exclusively
pathological meaning. It appears occasionally in later writers,
and to this day it has not, after all, lost this original meaning. It
is otherwise with Glisson, for whom irritability is a physiological
property and irritation a process of life in general dependent on
the natural properties of living matter. Thus he was led, through
a process of "contemplation," to admit the existence of the *biarchia*, the "principium vitae," or the *biusia*, the "vita substantialis
vel vitae substantia." And in order to allow no misunderstanding

of his ideas to arise he expressly states that this is the *archaeus* of van Helmont—the *vis plastica* of plants and animals.[8]

In the course of these philosophical discussions, he wanders, however, into the same erroneous way into which, even in recent times, so many learned men and excellent observers have been enticed. This is the way of unlimited generalization. The human mind is only too inclined to make what is unintelligible in particular phenomena intelligible by generalizing it. Just as an attempt has recently been made to render consciousness intelligible by representing it as no more than a general property of matter, so Glisson thought he could attribute to the active principle (*principium energeticum*), which he believed to be present in all matter, the three properties of living matter that he considered fundamental, namely, the *facultas perceptiva, appetitiva et motiva*. All matter would, accordingly, be sensitive, would thus be stimulated to drives, and would move as a consequence of these drives.

It is not necessary for the purpose of our present inquiry to continue with these considerations, so much the more since they are quite contemplative in character (in the Paracelsian sense), and in their generalized form do not appear to be important in the history of the advance of knowledge.

What is alone of significance for us is concerned only with actual life in the narrower sense of analytic science. It was not the "principium energeticum" set by up Glisson, which stimulated his successors again to continue his observations, but rather the process of irritation which he described, and the fundamental characteristics of living matter on which it depended. In this way he became indeed the forerunner of a more exact study of life and of the properties of living matter.

Unfortunately, a misunderstanding arose at this point, leading his followers into a group of serious errors. Glisson, following here the example of van Helmont, was convinced that nerves contracted when stimulated. He combined this with the notion that, by contraction of the nerves, or even of the brain, the fluid contained therein was driven to the peripheral parts. This notion, shared by Willis[9] and many other physicians of that time, is the reason why irritability was identified with contractility. Even the great master Hermann Boerhaave,[10] and his pupil Gaubius,[11] the first writer on general pathology, considered sensibility and motility to be common properties of at least all the solid parts of the body. The former considered it proven that hardly a single part of the body did not possess sensibility and motility. Thus it becomes understandable how Haller himself carried the idea that irritability meant the same as contractility from his student days in Leyden to his chair at Göttingen. It was in this sense that he understood the irritability of muscles, and in the same sense he denied it to nerves.

The dispute over the irritability of muscles has continued into the present century; its long duration becomes intelligible only when we consider that, without precise understanding of its historical development, even the statement of the question is liable to cause misunderstanding.

It has been established that, as far as we know, the nerves are not contractile like the muscles; the muscles, on the other hand, are not only contractile but irritable. Irritability and contractility are not identical, even when they occur in the same part. The current in the nerves, alternatively, cannot be compared with the blood stream; it does not consist in the movement of a fluid, but is of electrical character, and hence there is no need for a contraction of the nerve-tubes in its production.

It was also an erroneous conclusion that every stimulated part contracted. Secretion, or, under certain circumstances, more vigorous nutrition, may occur in place of contraction as the final result of stimulation. Hence we use a more comprehensive term to express this final result, and call all of its forms "activities." While Glisson designated all *actio propria sic dicta* as *motus activus*, we distinguish different kinds according to the character of the effects or, otherwise expressed, according to the direction of the activity (nutrition, formation, and function); but we agree with the above investigator that every action is of an irritative character. In the stimulus, in my opinion, lies the *principium dividendi*,[12] with which we must distinguish between active and passive life processes, and in this way we also achieve a basis for a fundamental division of elementary pathological processes. How much work has been required to make this conception workable! And how great, even now, is the number of our colleagues who have not fully accepted it! The reason for this is twofold.

Most of the vital actions of life, however they manifest themselves in external phenomenona, are of complex character. As a rule, different parts, at times wholly unlike, each with its specific energy, combine to produce them. Not infrequently it happens that in the visible sum of effects one part behaves in an active, another in a passive, manner. Only the most minute analysis of the phenomenon, tracing it back to the elementary parts, allows the end result to be resolved into its components. Such an analysis cannot be expressed in ordinary language without great circumstantiality. No language in the world is rich enough to possess special expressions for every such combination. Only too often we extricate ourselves from the difficulty by regarding a complex phenomenon as a simple one, and by expressing its character in terms of some chief trait prominent in the general picture. This is the practical difficulty.

A theoretical difficulty is very often combined with it, however. The human mind naturally tends to examine phenomena for signs of their determining causes. The more complex the phenomenon, the readier is the imagination to convert it into a simple one, and to find a unitary cause. So has it been with respect to life, so also with respect to disease. The train of thought developed by Glisson is exactly opposed to such explanations. He had no scruples about dividing the unit of life into a large number of individual lives. Although the knowledge we now possess of the arrangements of the body was completely unknown to him, he nevertheless arrived quite logically at the *vita propria*, the elementary life of the separate parts. Admittedly this expression, as far as I can see, is not to be found in his works, but first occurs in Gaubius; Glisson, however, says emphatically: "Quod vivit per se vivit vitam a nulla creatura praeter se ipsum dependentem. Hoc enim verba vivere per se sonant."[13]

The unitary efforts of the subsequent period heedlessly passed over the work of which I have just spoken. Some returned to the old Mosaic dictum, "the life of the flesh is in the blood"; others gave the nervous system, in particular the brain, first place in their considerations. Thus was renewed the old struggle, which for thousands of years had divided the schools of medicine into humoral and solidary pathology. Even when I began to participate in scientific work, hematopathologists took a hostile attitude toward neuropathologists.

In England humoral pathology found strong support in the great and legitimate authority of John Hunter. Although this experienced practitioner never lapsed into the one-sidedness of the later pathologists, but also sought in the solid parts that "living principle" the existence of which he assumed, nevertheless in his investigations the blood, as its chief carrier, took precedence over all other parts.

One must bear in mind that Hunter laid special stress on the circumstance that life and organization are not necessarily bound to each other, since unorganized animal substances can also possess life. He started, as has already been mentioned, from the erroneous notion that eggs are not organized, and that it was only during hatching that the first act of organization, namely, the formation of vessels, took place. He considered a "diffuse matter" (*materia vitae diffusa*) to be the actual carrier of life, a material to be met with not only in the solid parts, but also in the blood. This matter was contained in the brain in a particularly high concentration, but it was in itself quite independent of all nervous structures, as the example of the lower animals which possess no nerves demonstrated. In the posthumous writings of Hunter, which Owen has collected, the very striking expression "simple life" is encountered, a state most clearly to be recognized in plants and the lowest animals. This simple life was in Hunter's view the ultimate source of all living activities, pathological as well as physiological.

Hunter was a thoroughgoing vitalist, but his materialistic, as it were, vitalism was completely different from the dynamistic vitalism of the German schools. If living matter could exist independent of organization, it was to that extent beyond the scope of anatomical research; but if it were present in unorganized parts, as in eggs, it must be the ultimate source of the organization which later appears there. To adopt a later mode of expression, it must be of a plastic nature. Here Hunter's views corresponded with those concerning the plastic lymph worked out by Hewson,[14] and it was only logical for Schultzenstein[15] to apply it next to the blood, and to designate the living substance present in the blood as "plasma." In this way the formative and nutritive processes of the physiological organism, as well as the plastic exudations occurring under pathological circumstances, could be ascribed to the same substance—seemingly a highly satisfactory result and one providing a most convenient basis for interpretations. Those adhering to this view did not hesitate to go one step further and to give this material of life a technical name; they designated it "fibrin." Evidently this did not quite correspond to Hunter's ideas, for no substance is known, either in the egg, in the plant, or in the lower animals, such as that to which he attributed simple life; but the needs of the pathologists helped them over all such scruples, and the plastic exudates were received as unequivocal evidence that fibrin possessed the power of organization. In the *crasis*[16] doctrine of the Vienna school, they were the bright spot of this latest kind of hematopathology.

Where fibrin was lacking, blastemas were installed. After Schwann gave the name "cytoblastema" to the formative material of the ovum, the way was open for assuming the existence of this ambiguously named material in other sites.

To be sure, the simple living substance assumed by Hunter was displaced by many living substances and thus the entire advantage gained by a unitary theory of life was at once lost.

Even when the cell contents were finally designated "protoplasm," and the one demand of Hunter, namely, that the living substance must be present in the individual parts, appeared to be fulfilled, a single specific substance was still not found. No one dreamed of regarding protoplasm as "fibrin," and least of all did anyone consider it a simple chemical body.

But the conception of the blastema reawakened an idea which had occupied men's minds since antiquity. If a plastic substance capable of organization was actually present in the body, then its organization would be the first reliable instance of epigenesis. The long-disputed problem of *generatio aequivoca* appeared to be solved. What Harvey had taught concerning unbroken descent through the ovum was temporarily forgotten when the theory of descent through exudation appeared. Several generations of young doctors were raised in this belief. I myself remember my epigenetic youth with considerable regret, and it has required hard work for me to force myself to recognize the sober truth.

Meanwhile the attention of others had been directed to the body tissues. Among these the nervous tissues, in particular the mass of nervous tissue in the brain and spinal cord, aroused the greatest interest, because of their importance.

Hunter had recognized the importance of the brain, and called it the *materia vitae coacervata*. It was easy to perceive that it contained no fibrin, but experimental investigation showed further that neither the brain nor the spinal cord was of equivalent significance throughout. The more accurate the experiments, the smaller became the region of the vital parts, in the strictest sense, until Flourens[17] localized it at one single focus, the knot of life (*nœud vital*). Was the unity of life found in this way? Not at all! The brain is neither more nor less vital than the heart, for life is present in the egg long before brain and heart are formed, and plants, as well as an immense number of animals, possess neither one nor the other. In the highly complex human organism the brain and spinal cord have definite effects on other organs important for life. Disturbances here may be directly followed by disturbances of other vital organs, and sudden death may ensue.

But the collective death of a compound animal organism no more implies the immediate local death of all its special parts than the local death of some of the parts is incompatible with the continued collective life of the animal. As has been quite correctly noted, in the death of a complex organism there is a *primum moriens*, a part which first ceases to live; then the other organs follow, often at long intervals, one after the other, up to the *ultimum moriens*. Hours and days may elapse between the death of the whole individual and the death of its parts. The fewer nerves a part contains, as a rule, the more slowly it dies; I therefore consider the process of death in complex organisms as the best exemplification of the individual life of the various constituent parts, which is, in turn, the first requirement for the investigation and understanding of life.

A long time, however, elapsed before it was possible to return to this starting point, and to obtain a sufficient degree of support for the doctrine of the *vita propria*. The attention of many observers was directed to quite a different aspect of the question. In the final decade of the past century, at the same time that John Hunter, starting from careful anatomical investigation and exact observation in surgical practice, worked out his idea of living substance, a new system of medicine originated in Scotland, the so-called Brownian system, based on quite different premises. Brown[18] also was a vitalist; he too constructed not only a vitalistic system of pathology and therapeutics but one of physiology as well, although the latter was of dynamistic character. It contains little of the exact anatomical fundamentals. It is limited, rather, to speculation on the forces of living organisms. One can partly understand how this happened, if the history of this extraordinary man is kept in mind. I cannot go into it further at this point, but the remarkable fact remains that two contemporaries, Brown and Hunter, worked near each other without any evidence in their writings that they were acquainted. Brown struck out on his own path, and pursued it without troubling himself about the rest of the medical world. And yet even his first work, the *Elementa Medicinae*, had the effect of an earthquake; the whole continent of Europe was shaken, while the physicians of the recently opened New World bowed under the yoke of his revolutionary ideas, and within a few years the whole face of medicine was quite altered. True, the triumph was short; Brownianism disappeared as it had come, a meteor in the starry heaven of science. There would be no reason to treat it further, had not its impetus stimulated other men to do useful work in science. This impetus lay in the fact that irritability, or, as Brown called it, "incitability," was reinstated as a theoretical starting point, and also the stimuli which set living substances in action, the *potestates incitantes*, were brought to the fore. In so far as stimuli produce a state of arousal (*incitatio*), or, as Brown called it later, excitement, they came to be regarded as the cause of health and disease, and even of life itself; for arousal, he said, is the true cause of life. But, as the degree of arousal stands in a certain relation to the strength of the stimulus, a state of good health was supposed to be possible only with a normal degree of stimulation, while an excess or a lack brought disease in its wake. Of course arousal is dependent also on stimulability, a certain quantity of which, in the form of energy, is given to every creature at the beginning of its life.

The division of diseases into sthenic and asthenic, according to the degree of vital force manifest in them, has never been abandoned since, though it has been less sharply emphasized— now more, and now less, importance has been accorded it. In Germany Schönlein,[19] in particular, made this distinction the foundation of his opinions on special cases of disease and on their appropriate treatment.

But the application of the Brownian principles to physiology has proved to be of far greater importance. If life itself were dependent on external stimuli, the still current notion of the spontaneity of vital actions would lose all significance. Certain stimuli would, rather, represent necessary conditions of vital activity, without which life could at best persist in latent form. Indeed, even for this latent life the question would remain open: How does it arise, and in what does it actually consist? Brown very cleverly avoided this ticklish question by drawing all attention to active life and to the stimuli which call forth this action. To speak openly, science has since then deviated little, if at all, from this guiding notion. Even today, we cannot say what latent life is. We only know that through external stimuli it can be converted into active life, and hence stimulability is considered to be the surest sign of life, not of course of general life in the sense of Glisson, but of the actual and individual life of particular living organisms or their parts. Brown correctly remarked that stimulability differentiates living substance "from itself in the state of death, and from any non-living substance." Nevertheless, neither irritability nor incitability, neither *irritatio* nor *incitatio*, explains the nature of living substance or the nature of life.

In Germany the physiologists, in particular, took up this question. Among the first was Alexander von Humboldt, who in various papers, especially in his celebrated treatise on stimulated muscle and nerve fibers, tried to answer it. In the end he held fast to the assumption of a special vital force. The majority of pathologists and physicians followed in his footsteps, and long and bitter controversies were necessary before, nearly half a century later, the belief in a vital force was destroyed. When du Bois-Reymond[20] described the electrical current in muscle and nerve in all its details, and at the end of his work demonstrated the inadmissibility of a special vital force, the venerable Humboldt formally and expressly renounced his youthful dream, with the exemplary submission of the true scientist to known laws of nature.

The hypothesis of a particular life-force had, however, neither positive nor negative value with respect to Brown's theory. Johannes Müller rescued for general physiology (where it has since kept its place) what was valuable in Brown's system, the doctrine of the integrating life stimuli. The external stimuli which produce disease have found their place in etiology; their significance has become the more sharply defined as we have learnt to distinguish more accurately between the cause and the nature of disease, a distinction which became more difficult as the *causae vivae* of diseases were recognized in ever-increasing numbers. And now a new task has arisen, namely, to draw into our sphere of observation the life of the causative agents themselves.

The way in which pathology has tried to approach the desired goal, to understand living substance in its diseased conditions, has taken us a great step forward. Pathological anatomy, especially, has opened this road. The more numerous its observations became, and the further it penetrated into the details of the changes, the smaller became the field of so-called general diseases. Even the first steps of the medieval anatomists had the effect of drawing attention to local diseases. In the first and longest period, which we may designate as that of "regionalism," the pathological anatomists sought for disease in one of the larger regions or cavities of the body—in the head, chest, or abdomen. In the second period, ushered in by the immortal work of Morgagni[21] shortly before the time of Brown and Hunter just discussed, they endeavored to find in a given region the actual organ which might be considered the seat of disease. On this foundation arose the Parisian organicist school, which held a dominant place in pathology until late in the present century. In this school it was recognized that neither the organ, nor even a part of it, could be the ultimate object of investigation. Xavier Bichat[22] analyzed the organs into tissues, and showed that in the same organ now one and now another tissue might be the seat of disease.

From that time on, the gaze of the pathological anatomist was directed chiefly at changes in the tissues. But it soon became apparent that even the tissues were not simple substances. Since the third decade of this century, the microscope had disclosed the presence of cells, first in plants, and afterwards in animals. Only living beings contain cells, and both vegetable and animal cells have such similarity of structure that one can thus demonstrate cells to be the actual material of organization. This conviction has become general, since our embryologists, especially Schwann, have brought forward proof that the formation of embryonic tissues is due to cells in the higher animals and in man himself.

In the fourth decade of this century the science of pathological anatomy had already begun to turn toward cells. These investigations soon encountered great difficulties. Many tissues, at least in their fully developed state, appeared to contain neither cells nor their equivalents. I have, however, been able to demonstrate them in those tissues where their presence appeared to be most doubtful, specifically in bones and connective tissue. At the present time we have come so far as to be able to say that every living tissue contains cells. We even go one step further, for we demand that no tissue be called living where the constant occurrence of cells cannot be demonstrated.

A still greater difficulty then appeared in connection with the problem of the origin of new cells. The answer to this question had been very much biased by the so-called cell theory of Schwann. Inasmuch as this trustworthy investigator asserted that new cells originated from unformed matter, from "cytoblastema," the door was thrown open to the old doctrine of *generatio aequivoca*, which afforded all partisans of "plastic materials" an easy way of reviving their dogma. The discovery of cells in connective tissue and related tissues first put me in a position to detect a cellular matrix for many new growths. One observation followed another, and I was soon able to voice the dictum, *Omnis cellula a cellula*.

And so at last the great gap which Harvey's ovistic theory had left in the natural history of new growths, or, more generally, in the natural history of animal organization, was closed. The begetting of a new cell from an old cell supplements the reproduction of one individual from another, of the child from the mother. The law of continuity of development in animals is therefore identical with the law of heredity, which I was now able to apply to the whole field of pathological new formation. I overthrew the last barricade of my opponents—the doctrine of specific pathological cells—by showing that even in disease no cells are produced for which types and ancestors are not normally found.

These are the fundamentals of cellular pathology. As they have become more certain, and more generally recognized, they have also become the basis of physiological thought. The cell is not only the seat and carrier of disease, but also the seat and carrier of individual life. In the cell resides the *vita propria*. The cell possesses the characteristic of irritability, and changes in its substance, provided they do not destroy life, produce disease.

Disease presupposes life. With the death of the cell the disease also terminates. To be sure, neighboring and even far-distant cells may become diseased in consequence, but with regard to the cell itself the susceptibility to disease is extinguished with life.

Since the cellular constitution of plants and animals has been demonstrated, and since cells have been recognized as the actual living elements, the new science of biology has arisen. It has not yet solved the ultimate riddle of life, but it has provided concrete, material, anatomical objects for investigation, whose structure and active or passive properties we can analyze. It has put an end to the wild confusion of fantastic and arbitrary notions such as I have just described; it has placed in a strong light the incomparable importance of anatomy, even for the finest processes in the body; finally, it has taught us the identity of life in the highest and lowest organisms, and has thus given us a priceless tool for comparative investigation.

Pathology also has its place in the science of biology, certainly a very honorable one, for to pathology we owe the realization that the contrast between health and disease is not to be sought in a fundamental difference of two kinds of life, nor in an alteration of essence, but only in an alteration of conditions.

Pathology has been released from the anomalous and isolated position which it has occupied for thousands of years. Through the application of its doctrines not only to diseases of man, but also to those of even the smallest and lowest of animals, and to those of plants, it helps to deepen biological knowledge, and to light up still further that region of the unknown which still envelops the intimate structure of living matter. It is no longer merely applied physiology—it has become physiology itself.

Nothing has contributed more to this than the lasting scientific bond which has existed for more than three hundred years between English and German investigators, and to which we add yet another link today. May this bond never be broken!

One Hundred Years
of General Pathology

(1895)

THE CENTURY WHOSE TERMINATION the Friedrich Wilhelm Institute of Medicine and Surgery intends to celebrate brought to medicine the greatest transformation that it has ever undergone. To pursue this transformation through the many branches of science that we group together under the name of medicine would be so great an undertaking that it would not be suited to the present *Festschrift*. The task whose accomplishment will be attempted here must therefore be more narrowly bounded; it will be limited to a presentation of the transformation in scientific fundamentals requisite for the development of all branches of medicine.

A change approaching this in magnitude had taken place only once before in the history of our science, when the old school of humoral pathology collapsed in the sixteenth century. More than two thousand years had passed by without an essential transformation of the basic viewpoint regarding the nature of disease. The repeated attacks of the solidary pathologists had passed by without touching the roots of the system, though not without leaving behind visible traces. The doctrines of the school of Kos[1] had become established in the minds of men, and their dogmatic development by Galen[2] had, with each century, become more and more recognized as the correct presuppositions of medical thought. Indeed, they dominated the popular viewpoint as well, to such an extent that they even attained the sanction of the ruling churches, oriental as well as occidental. In the Middle Ages the great Dogmatist was without cavil given the rank of a Father of the Church; his writings were missing from no monastic school.

It is no accident that this tremendous changeover occurred at the time when the reformation of the Church was stirring all minds to their depths. Vesalius[3] and Paracelsus[4] were no less fortunate in their attacks on medical dogmatists than Luther and Calvin in their battle against those of the Church. Indeed, their success was even greater, for there was no country that afterwards continued to grant the old humoral pathology a secure right of domicile. Both men are usually called medical reformers; in reality they were more, for they created a complete *tabula rasa*. Their achievement would surely have been called revolutionary if it had taken place in the political realm.

In the minds of later generations appreciation of this revolution has greatly weakened; this is probably the reason why it has been passed off as no more than a reformation. On the one hand, this is due to the circumstance that neither of the two men devised a new system that might have granted to belief-hungry students a substitute for the firmly wrought doctrines of the humoral pathologists. Vesalius limited himself to purging human anatomy of the errors of Galenism and creating a generally valid basis, elaborated in a purely scientific spirit, for a conception of the human being. Paracelsus, to be sure, went further, but his doctrine, which rested primarily on alchemistic presuppositions, even in the beginning lacked the security required for permanence; more and more of its statements proved untenable as more and more was learned about the composition of bodies during the transformation of alchemistry into genuine chemistry.

On the other hand, the necessity for some new kind of medical system could not be repressed. The first firm basis for such a system was believed to have been found a century later, when William Harvey demonstrated the circulation of the blood and thus taught us of a fluid that constantly streams through the body, reaches all parts, and influences them to a greater or lesser extent—thereby satisfying the demand for a homogeneous material common to the whole body and to all processes in it. The blood had been one of the four cardinal fluids of the old humoral pathology also, not in the sense of a self-sufficient and independent substance, to be sure, but only as one of the materials in the composition of the parts of the body. For it was normally found only in combination (*crasis*) with the other three cardinal fluids, according to the traditional doctrine of the school of Kos. After its individuality was recognized, however, the other fluids obviously had to move into the background; more and more they became mere secretions. But blood, too, is a mixture; it proved to be a complex rather than a simple thing, with a composition which could be changed by a variety of other substances. Thus it happened that its composition (*crasis*) and the changes therein (*dyscrasis*) very quickly achieved dominant significance, not only in the speech of the medical men, but even more so in their estimation. A new humoral pathology gradually took origin, the same one that has persisted into our own time.

It is obvious that the new humoral pathology has, except for the name, nothing in common with the old. And yet it achieved the same dogmatic significance. Frequently, people acted as if it bore its name rightfully, as if it were a legitimate heir of the old humoral pathology. In place of the humors the "fluids" were created, frequently quite arbitrarily; dyscrasias were supposed to originate from these fluids, but neither "fluids" nor "dyscrasias" were demonstrated by genuine scientific investigation. Almost without exception, they were products of fantastic speculation. A glance into the literature of the past century suffices to reveal dozens of dyscrasias which have now been thrown out the window altogether. Scabies dyscrasia might be mentioned as a particularly horrible example.

Harvey himself was guiltless of these perversions. As a genuine natural scientist he kept within the limits of factual observervation. One need only read his two great works, *De Motu Sanguinis* and *De Generatione Animalium,* to see the difference between him and his followers, iatromechanists as well as iatrochemists. With these masterful works, Harvey became the founder of experimental medicine in the field of animal organisms, and, first and foremost, the spiritual father of the science which was soon to be known as physiology.

The resulting transformation of pathology is bound up with the school of Leyden, and in particular with Hermann Boerhaave, the master who founded it in the beginning of the previous century. This universal man—who accepted professorships of botany, chemistry, practical medicine, and theoretical medicine in succession, and who won resounding successes in all these branches of knowledge—was the first medical man since the time of the ancient Greek priestly sects, one may truthfully say, to leave behind him a genuine school. So great was his fame that Albrecht Haller, his most distinguished pupil, could designate him *communem Europae praeceptorem*. Although he was not entirely free from touches of humoral pathology, and was often wont to speak of the humors, the basis of his viewpoint was a sober consideration of individual processes in the body, preferably taking note of mechanical relationships in good scientific fashion. When he studied the blood and its circulation, he was in the particularly fortunate position of being able to put to use the demonstration of the capillary circulation—made a few decades previously by Marcello Malpighi[5] with the aid of the microscope—and the minute investigations of his countryman Leeuwenhoek,[6] who had very carefully studied the blood corpuscles. Local processes—inflammation, in particular—occurring in association with the changes of disease were now for the first time brought into the foreground of interest. For a whole century Boerhaave's *Institutiones* remained the basis for the instruction of all medical men who worked in the natural-scientific spirit; his students, faithfully maintaining and developing the method, carried it to every part of the world.

Scientific medicine quickly expanded in their hands. But the task of reconstruction immediately proved to be so great that, since his time, no similarly universal teacher has come forward. The students of Boerhaave divided the realm of the master among themselves. Two may appropriately be recalled at this point: Haller, who treated physiology, and Gaubius, who treated general pathology, as separate fields. They inaugurated the separation of these two disciplines which have since luxuriantly flourished. The *Institutiones Pathologiae Medicinales* of Hieronymus Davides Gaubius was the first textbook of general pathology which the world had seen; it remained the standard until far into our own century. The statement of Boerhaave with which it begins, *morbus est vita praeter naturam*, unmistakably indicates the completely altered point of view. In the language of modern science, the biological character of general pathology was proclaimed.

It may appear remarkable that the biological point of view arose so late in pathology. Hence I may refer to the Croonian Lecture, "The Place of Pathology among the Biological Sciences," which I gave before the Royal Society in London in the spring of 1893. I pointed out that the concept of life, though probably not much younger than humanity, was nevertheless pushed into the background during the era of the old humoral pathology. Hippocrates and his followers were content to speak briefly of φύσις, or Nature, without making an attempt to penetrate further into its character. Paracelsus first sought to define more precisely the relation of *physis* to life; developing the Arabian conceptions transmitted to him, he devised for life a special *spiritus*, which was supposed to differ from matter. He called this the *archaeus*. Every individual living part of the body—he fully recognized the *vita propria* of the parts—possessed its particular *archaeus*, and above all of these he placed the universal power, the *archaeus maximus* or *spiritus rector*, which governed the common life of the organism.

Thus Paracelsus laid the foundations for two different ways of regarding things. He revived the belief (basically a folk belief) in the individual life of the parts, but since he drew no important practical consequences from it the notion itself was very quickly lost to science, only to win power and significance again after several centuries. On the other hand, Paracelsus created a ruling instance of an entirely spiritualistic character in the *archaeus maximus*, which was supposed to exist independently of material substance, and to characterize and govern it in its workings. Owing to the inclination toward mysticism characteristic of the time, this idea found numerous adherents, nearly each one of whom passed it on in a new form, most frequently modified by some kind of iatrochemical addition. A few, among them the widely known van Helmont, held firmly to the *archaeus* as such. Others abandoned a more or less considerable portion of the whole conception, but retained the mystical core for a spiritualistic system. Whoever pursues the presentations of these later physicians to the end will realize that in spite of all seemingly philosophical or even physical disguise the *spiritus rector* is regarded as a real power.

A contemporary of Boerhaave, Georg Ernst Stahl, the renowned professor at Jena and later at Halle, went furthest in putting the mystical trappings aside. The system of animism takes its origin from him. In place of the *archaeus* he put the psyche (*anima*), which was supposed not only to form the body but also to determine all of its actions, and further, in accordance with circumstances, to eliminate disturbances—simultaneously, therefore, a forming, moving, and healing principle. To a very great extent he assumed that individual actions had a motivated character; in his explanation of the effects of the psyche he went far beyond the boundaries of actual experience—occasionally with marvelous prescience, but frequently in an entirely arbitrary and unjustified manner. His book *Theoria Medicina Vera* aroused widespread attention and exercised many stimulating effects on practitioners as well, but it gave rise to the founding of a genuine school in only one place, Montpellier. And even this school has ceased to exist in our own time.

The failure is understandable when the more important writers of the eighteenth century are consulted. This leaves no doubt that the notion of a direct influence of the psyche on the material substrate of the body called forth reservations in the minds of many people in France and Germany, and gave impetus to attempts to find some other explanation more closely related to natural processes. The way had already been opened by Francis Glisson, a contemporary and countryman of Harvey, whose important place in the history of the development of theoretical medicine I discussed in my Croonian lecture. He was the inventor as well as the interpreter of the word *irritabilitas*, which he did not identify with contractibility as Haller did (erroneously) at a later date. According to Glisson, irritability is the chief property of living matter; one must return to it if the effective principle of life is sought for. This principle—the *biarchia* or *biusia*, as he calls it—is the real "substance of life." However, he is far from regarding it as something peculiar to the living creature: on the contrary he refers it back to a *principium energeticum*, supposed to be present in every substance. Thereby the first step was taken toward interpreting life in terms of physics.

Glisson did not pursue these ideas further, yet it was only a short step to elevate the "principle" to a "force." This took place in France in the course of the eighteenth century, owing to men of the school of Montpellier (Bordeu, Barthez, Charles L. Dumas);[7] the life-force (*force vitale*) was formally introduced by Richerand[8] at a later date. Irritability continued to retain its dominant position throughout. In Germany, it was mainly Haller who, on the basis of irritability, created the special discipline of physiology, although in the previously mentioned and partly misunderstood sense; investigation was thereby moved from the region of doctrine to the region of fact, in accordance with the principles of his great teacher Boerhaave. It was also he who taught that irritability was a common property of living matter only, thus opposing the too general view of Glisson. Since he made no direct applications to pathology, it is understandable that he also exerted no decisive influence on the physicians of his time.

Among these, rather, philosophical systems and physical discoveries had made their influence felt since the beginning of the eighteenth century. Descartes had already altered ways of thought in many circles. Every philosophical system that followed was reflected in the minds of a certain number of physicians. This became most noticeable toward the end of the period dealt with, when the forerunners of nature-philosophy appeared. Galvani's[9] discovery of animal electricity had at this time directed general attention toward the underlying physical phenomena of life. He did not, however, live to see the successful application of his discovery to pathology and therapy. The immediate efforts of the physicians were restricted rather to the construction of an idea of a physical life-force that could perhaps be coordinated with electricity or magnetism. A barren, highly unfruitful turmoil of speculation soon filled the market place of medical opinion, where the monstrosity of animal magnetism finally raised itself up. Mesmer's[10] paper on its discovery, and the resulting inauguration of a movement aimed directly against science and investigation, a movement into which even outstanding practitioners were drawn, dates back to 1779. It was an evil time, one in which the disputes of vitalists and magnetists almost completely filled the scientific market place.

Standing quite alone in the history of medicine, an event then occurred which completely confused the minds of men. In 1780 John Brown, a Scottish physician, published a book entitled *Elementa Medicina* which unleashed a real storm all over Europe and in a few years found enthusiastic adherents in all countries. Brownianism disappeared just as quickly as it had arisen. Before the death of its founder (1788) a general sobering up had already taken place. Both the sudden rise and the quick decline are explained by the preponderantly practical goal that Brown had set up. Before everything else he wanted to cure diseases, and he gave very simple and easily comprehensible directions toward this end. But practical experience ruled against him, even though his theoretical foundations may have been well considered. Moreover, he stood entirely on the basis of the doctrine of irritability. He had developed this doctrine so skillfully that his theory concerning the integrating life-stimuli was adopted and pursued by the best physiologists. Also, there was no dearth of additional attempts to reform practical medicine according to his ideas; the so-called stimulation theory of Röschlaub[11] had as a consequence the transition of this notion into modern clinical medicine. For the first time, people began then to speak of physiological medicine, but it was a long while before the mistrust which the collapse of Brownianism had awakened was stilled.

Meanwhile salvation from the endless battle of systems had

come. This we owe to a new science, pathological anatomy. To this science can be ascribed the merit of having directed medicine to the path of genuine natural knowledge for the second time— as Vesalius had done with "normal" anatomy for the first. I have fully developed the memorable course of this transformation at the Medical Congress in Rome; at this point, therefore, I can be quite brief. Giambattista Morgagni (died 1771) published his epoch-making book *De Sedibus et Causis Morborum* in the year 1761. It included the abundance of observations that he and his teacher Valsalva had collected in a careful and detailed manner over a long period of years, together with a comprehensive presentation of all the pathological-anatomical data that were widely scattered through the literature. It was the first time that the entire sum of factual knowledge concerning the material changes caused in the body by disease had been presented to the world. The result was impressive. Almost more than in Italy even, the effect made itself felt in England, France, and Germany. Pathological anatomy became the basis of pathology generally, and medicine was elevated to the rank of a natural science.

In England it was especially John Hunter (died 1793), a highly regarded surgeon, who recognized the significance of pathological anatomy. To him we owe the founding of the first great museum of pathological preparations, one which has become the prototype of the many continental institutions of the same kind. Doctors and students were thus afforded the invaluable opportunity of becoming acquainted, through the autopsy, with the changes on which practical or (as we now usually say) clinical activity ought to rest. Only since that time have we become accustomed to follow and interpret, in the manner of the natural scientists, the material processes of disease. John Hunter has still another merit, no less great. He introduced the experimental method into pathology, and henceforth observations on living animals were used for the correction and extension of anatomical investigations. On the basis of such experience it was possible for the investigator named to set up general doctrines of proven significance. These soon became the standards of general pathology in England, and maintained their rank into modern times. The Atlas of his student Baillie[12] (the first of its kind) appeared in 1793.

Such was the condition of general pathology one hundred years ago. I had to be rather detailed, in order to prepare the reader for a general evaluation of the progress that has been made in the past one hundred years (1795–1895). To this end it would perhaps be useful to repeat from previous pages the chief names and dates.*

Paracelsus	†1541	Bordeu	†1776	
Vesalius	†1564	Haller	†1777	
Harvey	†1658	Richerand	†1779	
Glisson	†1677	Mesmer	†1815	1779
Malpighi	†1684	Gaubius	†1780	1758
Leeuwenhoek	†1723	John Brown	†1788	1780
G. E. Stahl	†1734	John Hunter	†1793	
H. Boerhaave	†1738	M. Baillie	†1823	1793
Morgagni	†1771			

At the opening of the year 1795 anatomy and physiology had achieved firm foundations, pathological anatomy had just started, and experimental pathology was barely taking its first steps. One after another the great pathological systems had collapsed, and general pathology, hardly more than a generation old (thirty-seven years), was completely without a system. Special pathology, alone, not infrequently seduced its proponents into hazardous speculations and into the premature application of *a priori* credos to practical matters—seducing many students, and even many older but overhasty men.

Berlin had been relatively little influenced. In 1795 it had as yet no university, and the academy of sciences had only rarely dealt with matters of pathology. Representation from the field of medicine fell chiefly on the medical-surgical college, which had limited its instruction largely to practical tasks. The connection of the Charité hospital and its physicians with the military authorities in regard to teaching was of so much the more influence

* Dates without a cross designate the first appearance of the major work.

in view of the fact that the wars of King Frederick II had sufficiently indicated the importance of surgery. The names of Schaarschmidt, Eller, Pallas, Henckel, Schmucker, Bilgauer, Theden, and Mursinna have become known far beyond their fatherland. But internal medicine had well-known representatives also; it may suffice to recall Selle and Formey. None of these men, however, achieved a determining influence on medical theory. The merits of Johann Nathanael Lieberkühn[13]regarding anatomy, especially that of the bowel, and those of Gottlieb Walter[14] regarding a more exact knowledge of the bones, are unforgotten; the importance of Johann Friedrich Meckel,[15] the precise investigator of heart diseases, could receive no higher recognition than the dedication to him by the great Morgagni of the fifth book of his *De Sedibus et Causis Morborum* in 1761. In this connection it should be recalled that a native of Berlin, Caspar Friedrich Wolff[16] (from 1759 on), in a series of papers laid the foundations for that branch of investigation which soon afterward yielded brilliant results in embryology.

Disputed questions in pathology moved more sharply to the foreground precisely at the time of the foundation of the new institute. The vitalists were first on the scene. Already present in its infancy, the doctrine of the life-force was developed with rare skill and great acumen by two men who are particularly closely related to our subject. One was the sophisticated and experienced Johann Christian Reil, whose famed essay concerning the life-force appeared in the first volume of his *Archiv für die Physiologie* in 1796, and who was called to the new university in Berlin as its first clinician (working there for only too short a time, regrettably) after losing his chair at Halle; the second was Christoph Wilhelm Hufeland,[17] subsequently the royal physician, who published his *Ideen über Pathogenie und Einfluss der Lebenskraft auf Entstehung und Form der Krankheit* in 1795 as a professor at Jena. While Reil attempted to give the life-force a more scientific interpretation, and in this way arrived at the conjecture that it was a heightened galvanic process taking place in the various parts, thus representing a *vita propria* of the parts, Hufeland held fast to the idea of a unified force, common to the whole body, therefore a kind of *archaeus maximus*. In this way he drew nearer to the mystics, and it does not surprise us that, for a time at least, he was enthusiastic about Mesmerism. This error brought its own retribution, in the worst way, to everyone who submitted to it. The rise of Mesmerism was nowhere more important than in Berlin, where two chairs in the medical faculty and entry into the Charité hospital were granted it (by Director Kluge), and nowhere was its fall deeper and more disgraceful. Altogether, decades passed before even the height of the flood had run its course.

Meanwhile, other and no less abnormal phenomena had appeared, among them homeopathy, whose incomprehensible doctrines impressed many physicians and even more laymen. The *Organon der rationellen Heilkunde* appeared in 1810. Hahnemann, too, began with the life-force, which he designated as "purely spiritual"; disease was supposed to be of dynamic nature and thus not to be grasped by the senses. No conclusions for general pathology resulted from this approach; the entire theoretical structure of homeopathy, just as of its variants such as isopathy, was erected for therapeutic purposes. It should not be overlooked, in this connection, that Hahnemann exercised a beneficial influence; he was the first to test systematically the effects of medicaments on healthy people. However, his test methods were so peculiar that no scientific pharmacologist could follow them; thus homeopathy has extremely little to show in the way of positive results. It has prolonged its sham life into the present, but the course of science has thereby been neither accelerated nor, fortunately, delayed.

An inclination to mysticism is so deeply rooted in human nature that there is hardly a period in which it does not occasionally come to light. Educated men then sink back into a thoughtless state usually attributed only to savages. Nothing favored homeopathy more than the mystique of the minimal dose; originally greeted with some recognition as a useful corrective against the polypharmacy of the dominant school of medicine (called allopathy by the homeopaths) and its often enormous doses, the minimal dose later served only as a means of refuge for the despairing invalid, and as a plaything of blasé circles. Here homeopathy encountered animal magnetism—in particular the somnambulism which grew out of it—and the more the currently puffed method moved away from the known laws of nature, the greater was the fanaticism of its adherents. The period of "table-tipping" has shown us how many otherwise quite well-educated and knowledgeable men could be carried away, moved only by the confident hope that here a new and completely different natural force, marvelously having remained unobserved until then, had revealed itself.

It lies beyond the purpose of this presentation to review the further developments which the spirit of Man, lusting after the miraculous, has brought to light in the course of time. It would otherwise be pertinent to speak here of spiritualism, but this variety of modern mysticism, first cultivated in America, has had little success in Germany. In no way does it participate in the development of scientific pathology. No "spirit" has revealed a new law; the spiritualistic "mediums" are as intellectually barren as the somnambulists. Even the newest discovery, hypnotism—the latter-day revival of the ancient temple-sleep—offers little justification for including it among the branches of knowledge that teach basic principles. Admittedly, Germany was very much involved in its spread, almost as much so as with homeopathy, but its real homeland was France. Much of the dark side of the psychic life has thus been opened to observation, but nothing has really been illuminated. Least of all has the nature of the psyche been disclosed.

Still, it was a real stroke of fortune that spiritualism and hypnosis were born in the same period during which the methods of medicine were completely altered. Animal magnetism and homeopathy had arisen at a time when vitalism, particularly in Germany, still exerted almost sovereign power. The seed sown by Reil and Hufeland had grown into a luxuriant weed, tended by *Naturphilosophie*. From Schelling to Hegel, nature-philosophy had become increasingly bold in its *a priori* constructions; but no science offered doors more open to its inroads than medicine. The young knew least of all how to defend themselves from the seductiveness of abstract thought. When one reads the biographies of our great masters, it appears that hardly one of them did not begin as an adept of nature-philosophy. It may suffice to recall Alexander von Humboldt and his "rhodian genius,"[18] Döllinger, Philipp von Walther, Schönlein, and Johannes Müller. The entire world of scientific medicine stood under this spell in the first decades of the present century. It was the period of the so-called natural-philosophical school. Only with the greatest of difficulty and with the summoning up of all its powers was medicine able to guard against the onrush of Mesmerism and homeopathy.

The University of Berlin was founded at this time (1810). It was born under the heavy pressure of foreign domination; a few years later many of its faculty joined the uprising of the people in the wars for freedom, and took part in the restitution of the Prussian state. There was little time for scientific work. But even after peace had again been won, the situation was a very precarious one. Nature-philosophy held fast to its leading position, and instead of genuine work the comfortable method of *a priori* speculation spread ever wider into the true scientific disciplines. Only one personality successfully resisted the pressure of this barren erudition. Alexander von Humboldt, who, after his return from his long scientific journeys in America, had devoted years of strict analytical and experimental effort to make himself at home in every branch of knowledge, came into the closest association with King Frederick William III. More and more every year he became the acknowledged Maecenas of all natural scientists, even, one can almost say, of all scholarly investigators. At his instigation and with his help one scientific foundation after another was created, and one chair after another was filled with proponents of the new method. Thus was readied, as I expressed it in my inaugural speech as rector, the transition from the philosophical to the scientific period, and when the aged king closed his eyes in 1840 the transition was largely complete.

With respect to medicine the rebirth began when the chairs in anatomy and physiology were occupied by men who engaged in serious and persistent work as genuine natural scientists, who knew how to implant at an early period in their students the spirit of independent, objective observation. Our grateful recollections are linked to the names of Rudolphi[19] and his great pupil Johannes Müller. The anatomists of that time still occupied an immense field of activity and investigation; in addition to human anatomy they taught physiology and comparative and pathological anatomy. Thus their influence extended far beyond the boundaries of anatomy itself into the field of the pure natural sciences, as well as into the field of medicine. It was as if they had been officially established to present broad points of view, and to bring basic questions into the foreground of study. And they accomplished this task commendably.

But also outside of our University, and outside of our country, they found powerful support. It was primarily Johann Friedrich Meckel the younger[20] who started the movement in Germany. He accepted the chair of anatomy at Halle, and his investigations were always of an essentially anatomical character. However, he developed anatomy in two directions that have been of the greatest importance for pathology. First of all he took up the embryological investigations begun by Harvey, Haller, and Hunter, extending them to the development of individual organs and following these into extrauterine life. In so doing he encountered those numerous anomalies of development which bring about congenital malformations. From time immemorial this had been the exercising ground of unchecked mysticism. Nobody knew how to explain the occurrence of congenital malformations, except as effects of demonic powers if not of the devil himself. The ancients had already called such formations "marvels" (τέρατα, *monstra, portenta*). Natural scientists had passed them silently by, for the most part. Now Meckel discovered that even here an accordance with law was to be found; he showed how, under certain circumstances, normal development might succumb to abnormal tendencies, in which the typical form—its peculiarity traceable back to a number, frequently small, of irregularities (defects, excesses or disturbances in the arrangement of the individual parts)—could still be recognized; finally, he found in addition the causes bringing about defective, excessive, or atactic formation in many anomalies. Thus congenital malformations became comprehensible and teratology (the study of monstrosities) became a new member of the array of anatomical subjects. It is truly no exaggeration to say that the most obscure field in pathology was first illuminated for natural science by Meckel.

Even such a deeply sensitive, poetic spirit as Goethe was unable to escape from the temptation to see law in the multiplicity of forms of organic structure. Prepared by long years in the study of plant metamorphosis, he turned to osteology, and as early as 1784 had already discovered the intermediate maxillary bone in the human being, a discovery that was of the greatest importance for the interpretation of hare-lip. Soon afterward he became active in the investigation of the development of the animal cranium, and as early as 1790 he arrived at the vertebral theory of the skull. Not only the validity of his interpretation, but even more the merit of his claim to prior discovery has been much disputed up to the present day. Unquestionably, however, in pursuing these investigations and following the path of Caspar Friedrich Wolff, Goethe developed in an ever more clear-cut manner the genetic method of study which is currently looked on as foremost in the entire rank of biological disciplines. A sufficiently long time elapsed, to be sure, before it achieved full recognition in pathology.

This method was first fully accepted in pathological anatomy, and we may be permitted to claim for Germany the chief merit of having opened this path. It was the genetic grounding of teratology by Meckel which furnished the prototype for later workers. But the paucity of larger hospitals in the German states and the difficulty of carrying out autopsies limited our countrymen's opportunities in precisely the two practical fields most important to the exact study of pathological development, and the fruitful union of pathological anatomy with the clinic was frequently hindered. This explains why pathology on the whole made far more rapid progress in France and England, where there were numerous hospitals larger than in Germany, with no difficulties attendant upon their scientific use. The Parisian pathologists were extraordinarily favored, and thus the medical school of Paris as early as the end of the last century became the foremost in the world, at which even the English sought instruction. Until far into the third decade of our century it was counted as a special advantage for our young medical men also to have completed their education in Paris.

The history of the school at Paris is bound up with the name of a man who was just thirty-one years old when his life ended. Xavier Bichat, after he had begun his medical studies in Montpellier and finished them in Paris, started in 1795 to give experimental and demonstrative private courses in anatomy and physiology. In 1801 he received a post as physician in the Hôtel Dieu, and he threw himself with the greatest zeal into pathological anatomy. He too was a vitalist, but he rejected the idea of a unified, abstract principle, and, like Haller, turned to the investigation of the vital functions of individual parts. In this way he achieved the well-known differentiation of tissues, which he depicted in more detail in his general anatomy in 1801. His desire to base pathological anatomy, and thus pathology in general, on the doctrine of the tissues did not reach fruition. On the contrary, it was precisely his most talented pupils who remained with the organs, and with good reason the doctrine developed by them received the name of organicism.

However, even this rather limited doctrine was an indication of tremendous progress. For it represented the first consequent development of the "anatomical idea," which Morgagni had expressed in the phrase "seats of disease" (*sedes morborum*) and which reached far beyond the earlier investigations of regionalism. Exact investigation of the particular changes that the individual organs undergo in disease began with organicism; although organicism remained entirely macroscopic, it nevertheless furnished scientific, thorough, and accurate depictions of changes actually observed, and these depictions followed an exact terminology that could in turn be used for diagnosis as well as possibly for marking out the genetic course of the processes of recovery and disease. The great significance for practical medicine of this improved method quickly became obvious when two of Bichat's prosectors, Laennec[21] and Dupuytren,[22] were placed at the head of clinical divisions. The first carried out a reform of clinical instruction in internal medicine, the second in surgery; for decades their writings remained the common textbooks in which the norms for practical knowledge were sought. Many discoveries in clinical investigation, until then almost forgotten—such as percussion, already discovered by Auenbrugger[23] (*Inventum Novum*, 1761) —for the first time achieved general recognition, assisted partly by the much more important discovery of auscultation by Laennec (1819).

The influential activity of Magendie, who had applied the experimental method (1816) to an extent never dreamed of previously in shaping physiology in the form of empirical science, and who at the same time had introduced it into the course of instruction with a completeness not even surpassed in later years, began about this time. With him a thorough, pugnacious, and convincing—owing to his evidential proofs—opponent of vitalism entered the lists; if he did not entirely succeed in doing away with it, nevertheless he did remove it to some extent from the limelight. As he deliberately led general pathology toward the goal of pathological physiology, he won from dreamy speculation a place for objective investigation. The freedom of movement thus achieved was most favorably influenced by the progressive development of pathological anatomy, whose chief proponent, Cruveilhier, wrote the first real textbook on the subject (1818) and at the same time offered, in the best of the Atlases in color, a workable foundation for the general understanding of the most important changes in the viscera. Andral[24] then furnished a complete presentation of pathological processes in an outline of pathological anatomy (1832), and thereby created for almost all civilized countries a common basis for the evaluation of pathological-anatomical doctrines. A new phase of hematopathology begins with him; not only did he derive the majority of severe local processes from disturbances of the capillary circulation, following the school of Leyden, but also, together with Gavarret,[25] he strove to create a pathological hematology based on analyses—though not always reliable ones. When a school of physiological medicine formed close by, chiefly under the influence of Broussais,[26] the attempt to derive so-called general processes, such as fever, from local conditions of the inner organs became dominant there as well.

While the school of Paris developed and its influence spread, English medicine, supported by a great number of isolated hospitals and the medical colleges united to them, maintained its eclectic character. Many of the younger men sought their welfare in Paris, and Andral achieved almost more influence in England than at home. Credit belongs to various hospital physicians, and particularly surgeons, for having sought out independent paths of investigation. The experimental method attained new goals in their hands. High above the number of these experimenters tower two men who completely transformed the physiology and pathology of the nervous system: Charles Bell (1821), who with great acumen discovered the motor and sensory divisions of the peripheral nerves, and Marshall Hall[27] (1836), whose labors were in the broad field of reflex activity. The unforgettable merit of these men is not diminished by the fact that it was Johannes Müller who, by improving the methods of investigation, furnished conclusive proof of the accuracy of their statements—entirely apart from the fact that he simultaneously developed the doctrine of reflex activity independently of Marshall Hall. With this development, exact scientific investigation began to be fruitfully applied in the field of neuropathology.

During a great part of the period just described, in the first decades of the century at least, German scientific medicine still lay under the spell of vitalism, whose unfruitfulness became more and more obvious in the later days of its domination. This time the opposition of the younger men rested chiefly on the biological branches of natural science: botany and zoology. Goethe's industrious studies of the metamorphosis of plants, and Blumenbach's[28] expositions of the formative drive (*nisus formativus*), continued to raise new questions about developmental history in general and that of man in particular. Nature-philosophy tried to answer these questions, but for the most part with no success. In spite of this it should be recognized that the nature-philosophers, when their speculations were actually supported by ob-

served facts (as Oken's[29] were, for example), turned with unmistakable acumen in a direction first elucidated a half-century
later by Charles Darwin. Embryology was the only field in which
objective investigation had early attained security and success.
Thanks to the trail-blazing labors of Caspar Friedrich Wolff, it
had prematurely wrested itself free from the natural-philosophical point of view; in the school of Würzburg, owing to Döllinger[30] (1803) and his pupils, among them Carl von Baer[31] and
Schönlein, it achieved complete security and wide fame. Here
exact investigation was pursued, in a way that has since been
adopted by the entire world, by a master who had worked his
way free from nature-philosophy with his own strength.

It is therefore no accident that precisely in Würzburg the
basis of the pathological point of view and the methods of investigation as well as of instruction were suddenly raised to the
peak of modern science. I attempted to discuss this remarkable
development in detail in my Memorial Lecture of 1865 for
Johann Lucas Schönlein. We owe it to this man that everything
achieved by the school of Paris was introduced into the German
clinics: precise investigation of the sick by percussion and auscultation, pathological-anatomical investigation of the internal
organs, reliable epicrises, and the evaluation of individual cases
with a view to building up genetic knowledge of the nature of
disease. In addition came the first—albeit hesitant—attempts to
apply the microscope, chemical analysis, and physical instruments
to the profit of the clinic. Numerous students filled the lecture
halls and soon filled the chairs of the German universities. This
school has been called the natural-historical in contrast to its
predecessor, the natural - philosophical. This designation, first
chosen by the Jena professor C. W. Stark[32] for the outlook he
represented, was passed on to Schönlein and his immediate followers, chiefly as a result of the not too happy attempt of the
master to discover a classification of diseases according to the
"natural system" introduced by Linnaeus into botany and afterwards into zoology, and required by Sydenham for pathology as
well. The essence of Schönlein's point of view was not touched
by this classification—which was taught, by the way, for only a

short time. However, the name of the school can be retained in order to designate the transition from the natural-philosophical to the natural-scientific attitude. When Schönlein, in 1839, received his call to Berlin, nothing of the natural-historical deviation of his younger days was discernible. Since I myself had the fortune to begin the study of medicine at just that time, I can testify that he was as observant, unprejudiced, and exact an observer at the bedside as one could possibly wish for. What could be more characteristic of this than his elimination of the essential nature of fevers or of *the* fever and as far as possible the substitution of well-confirmed pathological-anatomical views!

Unusual for a German clinician of that time, this esteem for pathological anatomy dates from a closer acquaintance with French investigation. Contact with Heusinger,[33] who, after having worked for a number of years as a physician in the German army of occupation in France, held the chair of anatomy and physiology in Würzburg from 1824 on, offered Schönlein a particularly favorable opportunity for learning of developments in France. Heusinger returned with not only more precise knowledge of the pathological changes in the internal organs in important "fevers," i.e. typhoid, but also an understanding of the doctrine of tissues (for which he introduced the term histology); and by comparative anatomical investigations, carried out with the aid of the microscope, he made some extremely valuable contributions. At the beginning of his activity Schönlein himself had undertaken a journey to Vienna, where Johann Wagner[34] had been appointed the first professor of pathological anatomy, and where the systematic performance of autopsies, started by Vetter,[35] was being eagerly continued. Similar activity was now started at the Würzburger Julius–Hospital as well, and the foundation for a pathological-anatomical collection thus was laid; the autopsies themselves were done by the young men, among whom Bernhard Mohr, my predecessor in this position, distinguished himself through his care and zeal.

The natural-historical viewpoint had led Schönlein to a comparison of the exanthemata with plant vegetations. Unger,[36] the outstanding Viennese botanist, had taken up the parallel with "plant-exanthemata," while he at the same time pointed out the dependence of the latter on botanical and other agents. In 1839 Schönlein himself first had the good fortune to discover in at least one instance (porrigo, tinea, favus) the actual dependence of a human exanthem on a fungus, thereby giving the impetus to a long chain of very important disclosures regarding parasitic plants in the origin of pathological states in men and animals. He began with the discovery, just made by Bassi,[37] of the nature of muscardine (a disease of silkworms caused by the invasion of fungi, common in Lombardy) and he studied it in numerous examples drawn from Italy; when he had convinced himself of the parasitic character of the disease, he immediately turned to the microscopic investigation of favus in man and discovered the fungus later given the name *achorion Schönleinii* by Remak.[38] Just as scabies (up to that time regarded as a prototype of humoral disease) was referred back to a mite, so here a budding fungus was recognized as the cause of a disease which had been held to be not only of humoral but even of hereditary character. Thus the first secure evidence of the parasitic nature of disease was developed.

The idea of the "parasitism of disease," however, had long since been introduced into pathology. Paracelsus had described disease as a positive entity, as a kind of life within life, even as a self-sufficient organism. In accordance with this conception, disease had to be a real substance (*ens*). The more this notion spread, the more disease took on an ontologic aspect in the minds of physicians. This way of looking at things found its plainest expression in C. W. Stark, who flatly called disease a parasite, a "life-process that often bears in itself essential features of life." Thus the doctrine had appeared in the natural-historical school even before Schönlein, but it achieved its greatest significance in the work of one of his pupils, Ferdinand Jahn,[39] who defined disease as "a self-sufficient, lower life-process and organism; a pseudo-organism." Not a few of Schönlein's other pupils accepted this conception, and it is understandable why Wunderlich[40] (1842), one of Schönlein's most serious opponents, sharply attacked the natural-historical school in general and its leader in particular. To what extent he was in the right on the latter count may be passed over; in any case at a later time, in particular while in Berlin, Schönlein showed no trace of ontology.

Attention must be drawn to the fact that the "parasitism" of the natural-historians had nothing at all to do with later developments in the doctrine of fungus diseases. The idea of particular, parasitic disease entities is without doubt ontological in an outspoken manner; in the later conception of diseases caused by parasitic organisms, however, the parasite is not the disease itself but only its cause. The parasite was therefore not the disease but some organism foreign to the body, which (to speak with Stark) lived "on, in, and with" the body. As long as pathogenic microorganisms remained unknown, skepticism concerning the nature of the "parasites" of the time was hardly possible; the hopeless, never-ending confusion, in which the ideas of being (*ens morbi*) and causation (*causa morbi*) have been arbitrarily thrown together, began when microorganisms were finally discovered. Repeatedly, I have sought to separate these basic ideas from each other, though with little success. And yet one would suppose that nothing could be more simple than to draw a line between etiology and pathological anatomy—for this is what is involved. I shall return to this matter at a later point; here suffice it to say that, in my view, the disease entity is an altered body-part, or, expressed in first principles, an altered cell or aggregate of cells, whether tissue or organ. In this sense I am a thoroughgoing ontologist, and I have always regarded it as a merit to have brought the old and essentially justifiable requirement that disease should be a living entity, and lead a parasitic existence, into harmony with genuine scientific knowledge. For every altered part of the body has, indeed, a parasitic relationship with the otherwise healthy body to which it belongs, and it lives at the expense of this body.

The attacks on the ontology of Schönlein and his school, therefore, would not have been justified if there had been clear conceptions of life and disease at that time. Wunderlich, as a proponent of physiological medicine, opposed the pathologists of the time, but he accomplished nothing of significance for the theory of life and its individual activities; in fact, he did not even understand the new movement. One must bear in mind that vitalism persisted for a long time in medicine and that physiology, as it gradually disentangled itself from vitalism, sought above all for physical solutions. Admittedly such a goal hovered before the vitalists, but they believed themselves able to reach it by the path of mere speculation. It would lead me too far afield to examine in detail the sorry errors into which people fell. I shall limit myself to one which caused an unbelievable amount of damage. After Görres (1802) sought and boldly defended a "new basis of the laws of life in dualism and polarity," almost every pathologist believed it possible to derive the secret of diseased life from a disturbance of polarity. Thus the dangerous pseudophysical attitude won more adherents, and finally nothing remained other than to "devitalize" the life-force in general. The final destruction of the doctrine of the life-force was accomplished by Hermann Lotze,[41] the first physician for a long time who was also recognized as a philosopher.

General pathology had led, if one may so phrase it, a kind of still-life beside clinical pathology. At the time I myself became a student at the medical-surgical Friedrich Wilhelm Institute in 1839, the famous medical historian J. F. C. Hecker[42] occupied the chair of general pathology both there and in the university. Our textbooks were those of Gaubius and of the Viennese professor Philip Carl Hartmann (*Theoria Morbi seu Pathologia Generalis*, 1814). Hecker loved to conduct our recitations in Latin, therein offering a complete contrast to Schönlein, who gave the "Latin clinic" in the German tongue. Gaubius and Hartmann, as well as Hecker, were sober men, fortunately, and although something of vitalism and "idealism" remained with them, on the whole they were proponents of objective knowledge. What they lacked was an investigative path of their own, and what made them strong was an eclecticism that did not even reject the humoral-pathological doctrine of the "fluids." In any case, they offered nothing new and of significance; and therefore the attention of the young turned, with constantly increasing interest, toward the innovations of the newly arisen school of Vienna.

In Austria, too, it did not take long before work started in the direction pointed out by Morgagni. The older Viennese school itself (whose history Hecker has written in his careful manner, and whose period he limits to between 1745 and 1785) had not arisen on the basis of indigenous investigation. As this expert expressed it, it was a "transplantation of Boerhaave's school to Vienna, soon after the death of its originator." Gerhard van Swieten,[43] one of the most outstanding of the Leyden group, was called by the Empress Maria Theresa as personal physician and professor in 1745, and very soon he was entrusted with the re-organization of teaching and of the whole medical system. The most important fruit of this reorganization was the founding of the general hospital, which, to be sure, still had to wait many years for its opening (1784) by the Emperor Joseph. But in the clinical teaching establishments which van Swieten set up, a home was prepared for practical medicine as well as for pathological anatomy. From here new pupils continually went out into the wide domains of the empire. Clinical as well as pathological-anatomical instruction could now be developed in the grand style. This first took place in relation to the clinic, through de Haen,[44] who was called with van Swieten, and who also, after the latter's death, took his place. Owing to a remarkable aberration, however, this man had developed not only into a scientific investigator but also into a mystic! With the fanaticism of a monk, he defended magic and miracles, and opposed philosophers as atheists. He prepared the ground from which animal magnetism and somnambulism soon sprang up. What contraries in one man! The same physician who introduced the thermometer into the observation of the sick, and the autopsy into clinical investigation, believed in witchcraft, and persecuted witches!

Not until the time of Maximilian Stoll[45] did the clinic at Vienna again attain the peaceful and prudent character that had characterized the arrangements of the school of Leyden. But only for a short time did this gifted physician achieve real influence on the course of studies; in particular he did not succeed in elevating anatomical investigation, the importance of which for the clinic he fully recognized, to an independent status. Thus is explained the fact that the learned Eble[46] in his *Versuch einer pragmatischen Geschichte der Anatomie und Physiologie vom Jahre 1800–1825* (Vienna, 1836) could not name a single prominent Viennese pathological anatomist; only in passing did he mention Biermayer and Vetter. All of Stoll's pupils whose names history has preserved were one-sided humoral pathologists.

More than a generation passed before the new Viennese school documented its existence in the outside world. A product of the long, faithful labor of native Austrians, it had grown up almost in silence. But then, fully equipped, it suddenly came to the fore—under the leadership of two men whose fame soon filled all of middle Europe. These were Skoda, the internist who surpassed the successes of Laennec in auscultation and percussion, and, above all, Carl Rokitansky, the professor of pathological anatomy and the successor of Wagner. His famous textbook of pathological anatomy appeared piecemeal from 1842 on, immediately proving itself the best of all available textbooks in this discipline and the real basis of practical medicine. Without any reservations, one may designate it the finest flower of organicism. For it went far beyond Cruveilhier's textbook in the masterful vividness and precision—equal to the classics of the descriptive natural sciences—of its depictions of particular organ diseases, as well as in the richness and trustworthiness of its author's personal observations. Even today it remains unequaled.

But Rokitansky was not satisfied merely with writing a descriptive pathological anatomy. The last part of his three-volume work was devoted to general pathological anatomy, and therefore was essentially of a general-pathological character. The author—saturated through and through with the significance of his craft—also made no secret of his opinion that everything worth knowing in pathology was contained in pathological anatomy. He did not hesitate to put all possible local processes on this basis, and to construct a system of general pathology as well. This system was a reconstruction of the doctrine of crases—not, of course, in the sense of the old humoral pathology, but as a further development of Andral's hematopathology. Rokitansky depicted the changes in the composition of the blood with respect to chemical peculiarities at first, but he soon recognized that these, as far as they could be studied with the methods of analysis then available, did not suffice to explain all the characteristics of disease. At this point he fell back on a remedy of despair, that of increasing the number of known constituents of the blood (namely, fibrin and albumin) by assuming particular modifications resulting from various diseases. Pathological albuminates appeared admissible to him as the basis for different disease processes. Thus the path was open to a new kind of mysticism, for in the evaluation of findings the names of substances unknown and inaccessible to analysis were included among the names of known substances. With these hypothetical substances in the composition of pathological blood he constructed a group of blood dyscrasias from which the substances—separated off by exudation—were "localized." As far as the interpretation of local changes was concerned, exudates thus moved into the front line of consideration.

It should not be overlooked that, since the end of the previous century, a kind of "exudation" had already won a prominent position in the minds of physiologists and pathologists. English investigators (John Hunter and Hewson in particular) had attributed to fibrin the significance of a basic living substance. The "plastic lymph," according to them, represented the material for almost all formative processes in the body. Fibrin was soon proclaimed to be in addition the real nutritive material of the tissues, and when our general pathologist C. Schultz-Schultzenstein reserved the name "plasma" for the fibrin-containing fluid of the blood (*liquor sanguinis*), the great riddle of all formation and nutrition seemed solved. This notion of "plasma" was also a basic conception in Rokitansky's humoral pathology, for it also contained albumin, the second substance requisite for the scheme. Both substances, fibrin and albumin, with their unquestionably great variability, readily permitted the assumption of an arbitrarily large number of very different modifications, the so-called dyscrasic substances.

This double aspect of the new Viennese pathology then became the hallmark of the immediate future. On one hand, the strict natural-scientific pathological-anatomical depiction of disease; on the other, speculative constructions in basic pathology forming all sorts of arbitrary patterns. There was something that recalled the mixture of naturalism and mysticism of old de Haen. But the confidence of the master helped the pupils to fight down their scruples; the literature moved carelessly along the path of crasiological willfulness.

For a long time our university remained closed to the new school of thought. Johannes Müller, whose teaching assignment also included pathological anatomy, remained at a distance from the innovations, since—true to the custom of the German anatomists—he excluded from his field of investigation and teaching those fields pertaining to clinical medicine. Nevertheless, the clinical branch developed somewhat more strongly in the prosectorship (first invested in Phoebus[47] and later in Robert Froriep[48]) at the Charité hospital. Both of these outstanding men, however, modestly confined themselves to the investigation of individual cases proffered them. The great stimulus brought about by the occurrence of the first cholera epidemic had no lasting effect, and young medical men who wanted further instruction found themselves obliged to go to Vienna, in order to draw on the rich resources of the school there.

My own participation in the prosectorship occurred at this time. By 1844 the task of making the microscopical and chemical investigations required by the directing doctors and clinicians (with the exception of Schönlein) had been given to me by the military medical administration; simultaneously I was appointed assistant to Froriep. In this position I had abundant opportunity to make extensive pathological-anatomical investigations, and I was soon requested by younger friends to give a course as well. When Froriep left Berlin in 1846 I was made prosector of the hospital, at his suggestion. In the same year L. Traube began editing the *Beiträge zur experimentellen Pathologie,* the first undertaking of this character attempted in Germany—unfortunately broken off rather quickly. My essay concerning the plugging of the pulmonary artery and its consequences appeared there, as well as Benno Reinhardt's work on the origin of the microscopic elements in inflammatory products. A large field of pathology was attacked in an entirely new fashion. But the material in our hands grew so abundant that Reinhardt and I decided in the following year to found a larger journal with more ambitious goals. This was the *Archiv für pathologische Anatomie und Physiologie und für klinische Medicin,* first issued irregularly, later regularly, and finally in monthly numbers; the exclusive editorial supervision has fallen to me since the premature death of my friend and faithful collaborator. From 1847 to the present time one hundred and forty volumes have appeared—constituting one of the richest collections of pathological reports based on the natural-scientific idea, and at the same time a reflection of the immense activity that has taken place in this field in Germany.

It was a binding requirement that this work had to be carried out with constantly improved and more elaborate tools, primarily by making use of the microscope, since anatomy as well as physiology used such instruments and owing to Ehrenberg[49] the microscope had become widely popular. The transformation began in two disciplines, general anatomy (histology) and embryology, which must be considered the necessary basis for all further explanations of processes in human beings. With respect to the first, thanks to the activity of Purkinje and Valentin[50] a group of important investigations of the various tissues (among which nerve and bone tissue may be mentioned) originated in Breslau in 1835 with the discovery of ciliary movement. Johannes Müller had already published a paper, his *Habilitationsschrift,* on embryology at Bonn in 1830, and immediately afterward he developed laws of formative sequences in the genitalia, valid for all time and of the greatest importance for anatomy. In Berlin he turned his attention especially toward cartilage, bone, and connective tissue (first so called by him), the composition of which he also studied chemically. His prosector Henle joined him and in 1841 published a large textbook of general anatomy which served as a guide to all aspiring young men for the next decade. The number of men who worked in embryology then and in the immediate future is so great that they cannot be introduced in this outline, even by name. From the Berlin school Schwann, Reichert,[51] Remak, and Waldeyer[52] stand out. In Würzburg, Albrecht Kölliker[53] took the lead; the long list of his general-anatomical and embryological investigations brought great benefits to medicine. It was he who, in almost definitive fashion, taught us of the extent of smooth muscle in the body, particularly in the vessels, and who summed up all progress in microscopic anatomy with a sure critique, in his *Handbuch der Gewebelehre* (1852 ff.).

Decisive for that generation was the revolution in the conception of the origin and structure of living creatures, which in cursory presentations is usually rather too simply linked with the names of Schleiden (1838) and Schwann (1839). For there are many questions, fundamentally independent of each other (but nevertheless bound together in many ways), which had to be solved here, and in the solution of which they and other workers participated in different ways. At this point a brief treatment must suffice.

The first question was that of spontaneous generation. In spite of the weight of Harvey's authority—which had not extended over the zoological realm, let alone the whole realm of life—the idea of *generatio aequivoca* (epigenesis) repeatedly came to the fore. The smaller the living organisms revealed by the microscope, the more probable to many people seemed the idea that such beings could originate from a fresh creative act. A decision concerning this question had unusually great significance for pathology. Since nature - philosophy, still in its last flowering, also regarded spontaneous generation favorably, it thus became, particularly in relation to etiology, a thoroughly serious and practical matter to find out whether at least the lower animals and plants might arise without forebears. Such an interpretation suggested itself for many of the entozoa, where no one knew anything of reproduction—where, indeed, no one could even discover sexual organs. I recall the cysticerci and trichinae, the origins of which were still unknown at a time when I already occupied an established professorship. However, I was already an opponent of spontaneous generation at that time on general theoretical grounds, and factual proof with respect to entozoa was first brought forward by application of the experimental method—specifically, for cysticerci and tapeworms by C. Th. v. Siebold,[54] and for trichinae by Leuckart[55] and me. No less difficult was the explanation—even more laborious since it was not possible to draw a line between the plant and animal kingdoms—of the origin of the smallest organisms, a point of great importance on which even the industry of Ehrenberg shattered. Built up with so much care, his system of the infusoria—all of which he had taken to be animals—was negated in important parts even while he was alive, as large divisions of it were allotted to the plant kingdom: in particular, all that has recently (to be sure, without justification) been given the general name of bacteria. Organs of reproduction are not found in these creatures either.

Indeed, it seemed that nothing else remained other than to accept generation without parentage for such creatures. In the popular interpretation, which has persisted down to our day, they were said to arise from decaying organic substances, from the filth of houses, of swamps, and of the body itself. Even in pathology, intestinal worms had for millennia been thought to originate by spontaneous generation from the filth of the bowel (the "saburra"), and when in our day the microorganisms of fermentation and decay were more precisely described (the former by Schwann) the old idea came up again, the more strongly since the wide distribution in water and air of such organisms supported the idea of general decomposition. The natural - philosophical school even developed the idea that body tissues were transformed into minute organisms in the course of breakdown; a few of the boldest adepts of this school even believed that it was permissible to recognize in this process a naturalistic expression of the immortality of the life-principle. Step by step, these fancies were slowly repressed. Eilhard Mitscherlisch has the merit of having confirmed the reproduction of the fermentative fungi by continuous observation of them under the microscope, after convincing himself of the dependence of fermentation on certain fungi, and of decay on bacteria, respectively. Louis Pasteur, in a long series of delicate and careful experiments, has finally given a conclusive answer for the whole field of micro-parasitic processes.

Thus was *generatio aequivoca* eliminated from the interpretation of living things at the present time. I say expressly "living things at the present time," for the question of the primal origin of organic beings in the developmental history of the earth has not been answered. This remains a question, and it is therefore not surprising when radical interpreters of the course of creation and the descent of living beings return to it again and again. But for practical purposes in the real world, and for pathology in particular, meditations about primal creation no longer have any significance; all parasitism is transmitted. We can follow the new parasites from generation to generation, not always, admittedly, according to Harvey's formula *omne vivum ex ovo*, but with the firm conviction that every living thing has a living ancestor. The possibly pathological state of living things in no way alters this conception; seemingly entirely "degenerate" abortions are either human, plant or animal, and have been begotten by real men, animals or plants.

The second question is that of the further course of development of the complete individual from the germ or egg. A sufficient answer has been given by innumerable investigations of particular cases, and it is unnecessary to go into details at this point. As regards human beings and the majority of animals, the answer is to be found in embryology. In continuity with numerous preliminary investigations Schwann proved that tissues are built up from cells. It has been the task of his contemporaries and of the subsequent generation to reveal more details of this process. Even now complete agreement among investigators concerning all points has not been reached. In particular, a circumstance of the greatest importance for the understanding of large parts of the body has remained controversial. It concerns the formation of the "tissues of the connective substance." Reichert has grouped together under this name a rather large number of tissues which control the form and cohesion of the body, in particular the genuine connective tissues such as tendon, bone, and cartilage; in addition I have included the mucoid tissue and neuroglia. In all of these tissues a substance differing from cells is present, either between the cells (intercellular substance) or, at least apparently, even in their absence. Thus it has been believed, ever since Schwann, that cells are present in the formation of connective tissue cells at first, but that they disappear in the course of further development and change into fibers. The controversy is too extensive to be fully set forth here; suffice it to say that in the end the mature connective tissues were regarded as acellular. My investigations at Würzburg have shown, however, that cells are present at all times, not only in connective tissue but in bone as well—cells, to be sure, that are often very small and difficult to find. In my opinion, the last link in our understanding of the arrangement of our bodies as a cellular organization was thus disclosed, and a firm basis was laid for a factual evaluation of physiological and pathological processes. Since the higher plants also possess cellular organization, a unified approach to the interpretation of all these processes is now feasible.

The third question concerns the manner of cell formation itself. The main features of "Schwann's cell theory," as the doctrine of the origin of individual cells set up by that famous microscopist is called, he adopted from Schleiden out of botanical developmental history. This theory chiefly impressed his contemporaries precisely because it was very closely connected with traditional forms, and because it seemed to demonstrate what had generally been suspected. Schwann began with the doctrine of formative substances. A certain accumulation of these he called the "blastema" and, in relation to the cells arising from it, the "cytoblastema." He supposed that the cells arose in the cytoblastema like crystals in a mother-liquor; he even took this comparison literally, and flatly called the formation of cells "organic crystallization." What was more natural now than to call the "plastic" exudates "blastemas," allowing cells to arise in them according to the schema of Schwann—a theory that first gained adherents on a large scale in the Viennese school? This "hour-glass theory," as it has been called, went on from this point to suppose that the nucleus arose as a result of the organization of certain parts of the blastema; a fine membrane (the actual cell) formed about this, and a quantity of cell contents separated it on one side from the nucleus. More details are unnecessary for the present consideration; the above contains everything essential concerning this theory of the formation of cells.

Further investigations have shown that cells are not formed in this way at all. In addition the necessity of a membrane for the existence of a cell has been successfully disputed; only the nucleus and the cell-body (earlier interpreted as the cell-content) are essential. The substance of which the cell-body consists is now usually called protoplasm, a term borrowed from botany that, if taken literally, easily gives rise to misunderstandings. Over the course of years, in one instance after another, I have succeeded in showing that there are no pathological blastemas and that the new-formation of cells from blastemas has in no instance been unequivocally demonstrated. Thus any analogy with crystallization (which is also sufficiently different in other respects) drops away. Observation reveals, rather, that all new cells are descendants of older cells, and therefore that throughout the entire realm of plastic processes no law of formation other than that of inheritance rules. Just as entire organisms (animal as well as plant) arise by way of hereditary reproduction, so do individual cells. What I was able to demonstrate in pathological new-formations is valid for physiological ones also, as the research of numerous other investigators has shown. Any difference of principle has at this point dropped away. The hypothesis of spontaneous generation is just as superfluous for the cells and the tissues arising from them as it is false and superfluous for the whole organism. It is the cells, with or without intercellular substance, which remain. They are the truly living parts of the body, and it follows by necessity that the unitary cell-theory of all animal and plant life must consequently rest on them. This holds also in pathology.

Justice requires us to mention that the question of whether life is bound only to cells is not entirely undisputed. Thus Heitzmann[56] defends the view that intercellular substance is alive, and Grawitz[57] has sought to prove, in partial correspondence with this opinion, that new cells can be formed from the intercellular substance. The first view might perhaps be sanctioned if it could be shown that protoplasm was different from the true inter-cellular substance. The second appears for the present to be an unnecessary interpretation of the smallest connective tissue cells, which are difficult to find, and for which the author himself uses the very appropriate name "slumbering cells." In the main, as I see it, the cell theory is not affected by these views.

The use of this theory for a pathology of cells had to wait for some time. The important work of H. Lotze (*Allgemeine Pathologie und Therapie der mechanischen Naturwissenschaften,* 1842) did not reach the heart of the matter; he was mainly concerned with the ill individual as a whole. His views, upheld more polemically than constructively, indeed succeeded in repelling the life-force and vitalism, and showed the necessity of a mechanistic treatment of living processes, but accomplished nothing for positive science.

The labors of Henle produced an incomparably greater impression. He had already moved close to medical questions in his *Pathologische Fragmente* (1840); not only did he further extend the theory of fever of his teacher, Johannes Müller, which rested on a consideration of nervous processes, but he also resolutely developed the idea that the old conception of a *contagium animatum* might be justified. A later era confirmed this idea, but he himself discovered no new facts to support it. He developed further a speculative view, rather, the justification of which he sought to present in the *Zeitschrift für rationelle Medicin* (founded in 1842 by him and Pfeufer,[58] a pupil of Schönlein) and in his *Handbuch der rationellen Pathologie*. The rapid advances in empirical pathology made by his contemporaries soon overtook him, and he turned back to the broad field of anatomy, in which he has harvested great fame.

Johannes Müller himself, in the freshness of youth, had meantime taken up the microscopic investigation of pathology. He did indeed find new parasites, though in fishes and birds; by 1838, about the same time that the foundations of the cell theory were laid, he began studies concerning the finer structure and the form of morbid tumors, in which, for the first time, the theories of general anatomy were applied. If, after establishing the peculiarities and properties of enchondromas and cholesteatomas, of fibrous and other tumors, he gave up the effort with sarcomas and cancers, the difficulty of the task and the desire to keep to the traditional prognostic viewpoint of the physician excuse him. In order to maintain the conception of "malignant" new-formations he sacrificed the histological principle that had so happily guided him in the classification of benign neoplasms. In his school, nevertheless, vigorous work went forward. The inaugural dissertation of Ludwig Güterbock,[59] *De Pure et Granulatione,* containing the first precise description of pus cells, may be cited as an example. It should not be forgotten also that his most famous pupil, Helmholtz, began his work as a teacher, as professor in Königsberg, in the field of general pathology.

The prosectorship at the Charité did not remain aloof from these investigations. Froriep too turned toward microscopical studies, and his pupil Gluge[60] even discovered those "tailed bodies" which soon caused so much mischief in the study of tumors, because neither their discoverer nor his followers noticed that they had simply focused attention on the cells of immature connective tissue. In addition the first studies of Gluge concerning the "inflammatory globules," which Reinhardt and I later learned to know as cells in regressive fatty metamorphosis, fell in this period. When I entered into my assistantship I was able to begin my microscopical work with the same instrument that had served in Gluge's investigations. With it I made my first important observation—concerning the "white blood" (1845)— to which were added numerous studies on the colorless blood corpuscles, at the conclusion of which I considered myself justified in saying, "I claim a place in pathology for the colorless blood corpuscles" (1846). This has been granted them to an increasing extent each year, so that at the moment they have moved into the center of pathological interest.

Rokitansky's *Handbuch der allgemeinen pathologischen Anatomie,* proclaiming the new humoral pathology of the Viennese school, appeared in 1846. It was necessary to protect science from this false pathology of the humors. This I did in a critical review published in the *Preussische Medicinal-Zeitung* in December, 1846. To my great pleasure Johannes Müller expressed his appreciation in warm terms to me, and it soon appeared that my brief essay had also had an effect in Vienna. The "crases" have not since appeared in the scientific market place. The last "system" of general pathology was buried with them.

We had now arrived in the age of scientific medicine. And we were free and independent natural scientists, adherents of no system and of no school in the old sense. Observation and experiment, the ancient postulates of science, had absolute power; every authority had to bow before them. With their aid I progressed beyond every kind of humoral pathology, without sinking back into a new solidary pathology. For the cellular pathology that I immediately began to construct treated blood and tissues in the same manner. The functioning parts of each were made the objects of study; the blood corpuscles, red as well as white, were brought before the judgment seat of science, just as were ganglion cells and the cells of tissues. The isolated attempt of Spiess to set neural pathology in opposition to cellular pathology was wrecked on the misconceptions of its creator.

It does not seem necessary to develop the basic principles of cellular pathology in detail at this point. They are easily available to everyone. This doctrine, which of course embraces a cellular theory of life in general, starts from the cells as the really effective parts of the body and the true elements from which all vital action proceeds. But since life itself is only expressed through action, the true task of pathology is therefore an understanding of these different kinds of activity and of their disturbances. It is therefore in no way a mechanistic science (in the sense of Lotze), but rather a biological science. The mechanistic course of the isolated living acts is in no way excluded; on the contrary, penetration into fine details is impossible without exact investigation of the effective mechanism. Physical and chemical laws are not suspended by life, as was taught until a short time ago; they only become effective in another manner, as occurs in a state of health. Furthermore, an otherwise absent or repressed power does appear in disease or convalescence; the substance that is the carrier of life is also the carrier of disease. Spiritualistic leanings are excluded. Nothing prevents anyone from calling such an attitude vitalism. It should not, of course, be forgotten that no special life-force can be discovered, and that vitalism in this sense does not of necessity signify either a spiritual or a dynamic system. But it is likewise necessary to understand that life is different from processes in the rest of the world, and cannot be simply reduced to physical or chemical forces.

Just as no other feature brings this peculiarity of life so clearly into focus as does the hereditary character of the transmission of life from one generation to another, so has the victory of cellular pathology been made most secure by proof of the hereditary character of the natural history of plastic processes, or, otherwise expressed, of the developmental history of new - formations. When it became clear that no cell arises without—as we say in this case—a mother (matrix) that is, or was, itself a cell, then the principle *omnis cellula a cellula* became the recognized hallmark of the biological cell theory. Blastemas have disappeared and matrices have stepped into their place. Aside from cells, there are no histogenetic or organopoietic substances.

This conception is expressly ontological. That is its merit, not its deficiency. There is in actuality an *ens morbi*, just as there is an *ens vitae*; in both instances a cell or cell-complex has the claim to be thus designated. The *ens morbi* is at the same time a parasite in the sense of the natural-historical school, not a parasite in the sense of the bacteriologists. We shall return to this distinction presently.

When I left Berlin in 1849 to follow the call to Würzburg, I already brought the main ideas of cellular pathology with me, but they were not yet sufficiently clear. Studies of the connective tissue and of the tissues closely related to it carried out during the next few years first permitted me to take a great step forward and to show that the body is composed of cell territories throughout. In such cell territories I recognized potential loci of disease. A theoretical conclusion was thus achieved in the investigation of the "seats of disease" begun by Morgagni—in a much finer sense, to be sure, than the great anatomist of Padua had suspected, but nevertheless in a consequent development of his "anatomical idea." From that time on, the altered cell territory had to be the starting point for every general pathological consideration of elementary processes. Since most diseases are not elementary processes, but combined processes in which alterations of several or many cell territories coexist or are grouped together, not only special pathology but also the doctrine of general disease requires further investigation of the involved cells or cell groups, and primarily, indeed, always an investigation of the site or sites of the disturbance, i.e. of the "where" of the disease, of the involved anatomical parts. This investigation is not to be carried out with the knife alone, according to the usual and peculiarly anatomical method; the utilization of experimental and clinical data is frequently required. To give a familiar example of this, the ordinary fibrinous pneumonia may be referred to. It is a frankly local affection, but at the same time it is so regularly associated with fever, a so-called general affection, that it was still numbered among the inflammatory fevers until the beginning of this century. However, we should not be misled by precise knowledge of the local course—any more than by the dissolution of the idea of essential fevers—into studying only one side of a complex process. On the contrary, the local affection is to be fathomed by means of pathological anatomy, and the fever by means of clinical observation or experiment. Since fever also may be traced back to certain sites in the nervous system, the "anatomical idea" still remains intact.

Under the impress of such considerations, I developed the cell theory further while in Würzburg. In the general section of my book on special pathology and therapy I have set down a comprehensive picture of my views at that time. The foundations of these views were in many ways improved and developed more fully in a group of lecture-demonstrations held before a rather large group of physicians soon after my return to Berlin. Detailed lectures concerning morbid tumors were added to these later (beginning in 1863), as well as numerous individual investigations of mine and my pupils. Of these I mention the pioneering studies of my assistant, von Recklinghausen,[61] on the motility of pus and connective tissue corpuscles (1863), and of Cohnheim[62] on the migration of the white blood corpuscles (1867), which so completely changed the theory of pathological exudates. If it were at the moment a matter of writing a complete history of further detailed investigations, a great number of papers would have to be enumerated, from here and abroad, such as no earlier phase of pathology produced. But none of these papers marked a regression into earlier doctrines, or an essential change in viewpoint. A thorough and detailed discussion is therefore unnecessary for the elucidation of the progress in pathology I describe here, especially since the work of foreign investigators has also turned more and more in the same direction.

The only important group to come forward with another conception—not uncommonly in an opposing form—has been that of the bacteriologists. Since Ferdinand Cohn[63] extended the name bacteria (not always identical with bacilli) beyond Ehrenberg's rodlets to include all possible forms of the smallest microscopically visible living things, and even made globular bacteria of cocci, bacteriology in ordinary discourse has come to signify practically what I grouped together under the designation of mycotic diseases. Sprouting and filamentous fungi must be content to be reckoned with the bacteria; other workers, to be sure, classify the cocci as fungi. Perhaps a more accurate terminology may once again be found; meanwhile there is nothing else to do except to adjust our understanding to one which is irrational.

All mycotic diseases have in common the fact that parasitic microorganisms occupy the focal point of attention. All investigations in this direction must, therefore, strive toward the ultimate goal of ascertaining the effect of these organisms and of elucidating their particular variety of parasitism. From what has already been said, it is evident that this kind of parasitism is something quite different from the "parasitism" of the natural-historians. In actuality what is involved here is the action, if not the penetration, of independent beings in the human body in such a way that henceforth two or more lives are present side by side. Thus we return to a scheme drawn up by Paracelsus, except that he interpreted the "parasite" as a secondary organization springing from the body rather than as an independent plant of external origin. In the apparent similarity of these two notions lies a temptation toward a state of confusion into which many superficial minds of modern times have fallen, a state whose dangers cannot be overstressed. In this state there occurs, as I have repeatedly explained, the confounding of a *thing* with a *cause*, of the *ens morbi* with the *causa morbi*. A genuine parasite, whether plant or animal, can become the cause of a disease, but it can never represent the disease itself. Nothing demonstrates the necessity of this distinction more clearly than the fact that parasites live in great numbers in the healthy body, and that in certain cases parasites that are supposed to act as pathogens (more precisely, pathogenetically) can be harmless. If these effects do not develop, e.g. if diptheria bacilli are found in the throat of a healthy child, then no disease and thus also no *ens morbi* is present. On the other hand, if an altered part of the body, e.g. a new-formation (tumor), is called a parasite (with the natural-historians), one easily arrives at the idea of two "parasites" in the same body: the *causa viva* and the *ens morbi*.

In a paper on the nature and causes of disease[64] I discussed these relations in detail, with special reference to cellular pathology. Later I defined the relation of the body to the pathogenic microorganisms as a battle between cells and bacteria. Yet, even before this, I repeatedly emphasized that we are not always dealing with microorganisms. Time and again in this connection I have pointed to the process of fermentation started by microorganisms, to be sure, but by microorganisms which are almost completely harmless to the animal organism; the noxious character of fermentation lies in the products, whether alcohol or acetic acid, of the vital activity of the fermentative fungi. In this sense, from the beginning I have held to the theory that harmful or frankly poisonous substances of purely chemical character can be present in addition to microorganisms, and that the disease arising in consequence of the penetration of microorganisms should not without further ado be regarded as a "fungus effect." In the same sense I singled out, for the first time, the category of the "infectious diseases" and gave an entire division in my large *Handbuch der speciellen Pathologie und Therapie* to them. Since then, a group of poisonous bacterial substances, which have been designated toxins, has been described (especially by Brieger[65]) in connection with the ptomaines already pointed out previously by Selmi.[66] The number of infectious diseases has also been significantly increased by new discoveries of pathogenic microorganisms, and it cannot be said whether or not still further discoveries will be made.

The past two decades have seen a great many investigations in this field. Presentation of these would require considerable space, and it would be impossible to give conclusive judgments in every case. The fact that the invariable presence of microorganisms has been demonstrated, and that we have experimental proof of their activity in a number of the most important contagious and infectious diseases, suffices to indicate the immense progress of natural - scientific knowledge in this difficult field, which as recently as half a century ago was still endangered by highly arbitrary assumptions concerning the causes and circumstances of epidemic diseases. It has not yet been possible to find pathogenic microorganisms for all contagious diseases; it has not yet even been scientifically established whether contagion exists in the absence of bacteria. It may suffice to recall rabies, as well as the numerous diseases of the neoplastic group (from the carcinomas and sarcomas to the enchondromas and myxomas), which behave quite like infectious diseases in their spread through the body. Meanwhile, it is understandable that here too the hope of finding the desired parasitic microorganisms persists—not only in the minds of optimistic investigators and youngsters reveling in dogma—and that every new development in our knowledge of independent organisms (as recently with certain protozoa) in pathological conditions leads to a largely arbitrary inductive broadening of dogmatic formulas. For the calm observer this activity is sometimes rather disturbing. But the great and consoling difference from the method of the earlier speculative and aprioristic pathologists lies in the fact that every step in the path of the modern investigator can be precisely controlled, and that even the greatest enthusiasts proceed from real things accessible to experimental criticism. The rich store of factual observations and the eagerness shown in the pursuit of even the tiniest creatures is certainly most gratifying in comparison with the barrenness and inertia which were the hallmark of etiological investigation one hundred years ago.

Strange to say, the most recent development in these investigations has led to a result which has brought quite unexpected success in relation to practice, but a kind of retrogression into long-forgotten formulas in relation to theory. Louis Pasteur, the same investigator who first clearly and precisely demonstrated the hereditary propagation of bacteria and their mode of chemical action, has also boldly undertaken to use products of contagious organisms for combating the diseases caused by them, and for immunizing the animal body in general against their effects. The long series of new attempts carried out by him—from anthrax in ruminants and cholera in fowls, to rabies—links up with the well-known method of Jenner, who introduced cow-vaccine as a protective measure against smallpox. Since these efforts are concerned in part with diseases in which pathogenic microorganisms have not been found, the notion of the "lymph" has once again won a certain degree of credence.

The well-known attempt of Robert Koch, the happy discoverer of one of the most important of the pathogenic bacteria, to obtain from pure cultures of tubercle bacilli a "lymph" that would produce immunity against and cure tuberculosis, led to a new path that has finally brought *serum therapy* into the foreground of practical interest. A very complex process—although one, to be sure, with a prototype in vaccinia—is involved here. Fluid from pure cultures of bacteria, containing their metabolic products (as one says now), is first introduced into the body of a healthy animal, perhaps directly into the blood, and after a relatively long time there is a change in the animal, recognizable in the constitution of its serum. It proves to be a *curative serum*, for it favors recovery from the corresponding disease and grants a relative degree of protection against its development. This has been shown in diphtheria particularly, thanks to Behring's[67] procedure, which is based on careful experiments. Hope for unlimited expansion of this procedure in the treatment of other contagious diseases is understandably widespread.

A conclusive judgment cannot at the moment be given. Nevertheless, for a long time no therapeutic effort has won greater acclaim. Much more difficult is the question of the theoretical significance of serum therapy for general pathology. Enthusiasts see here a final triumph of humoral pathology, although a humoral pathology quite different from any preceding it. The old humoral pathology cannot come into question at all, but only one of the later forms—hematopathology, to be precise. But the latter, too, referred either to mere quantitative changes in the blood "crases" or to qualitatively abnormal substances reaching the blood either from the outside or from the inner parts. Preeminent among these stood the putrescent substances, for decades the object of numerous experiments. The doctrine of putrid infections(septicemia) had gradually passed over into general knowledge; everyone assumed that putrescent substances exerted a harmful effect and sometimes caused new putrefactive processes in the body. But no one had the right to conclude from this doctrine that the tissues of the body—let us say the cells for brevity—could be disregarded, and that a putrid infection was nothing more than an abnormal condition of the blood. The blood only contains the cause of the tissue disturbance; the disease is not in the blood, but is rather the effect of the cause on the cells or tissues.

From here to curative serums is still a long step, for in this case the formation of new substances in the body is involved, and if these are also found in the serum this is still no proof—indeed, it is not even probable—that they have arisen in the serum itself without definite activity on the part of the cells, whether of tissue cells or blood cells. The solution of this question must be the next task of science. It will at the same time furnish a criterion for judging the necessity of altering the basis of cellular pathology.

For the present, cellular pathology has found a powerful support in the progress of our knowledge concerning the effects of tissue extracts. Here only the extracts of the thyroid gland and the pancreas need be mentioned. Separated from cells, such extracts display indubitably important influences on the tissues of other animals and human beings, and there is no lack of examples of straightforwardly poisonous action. This has long been known of fluids from glandular organs of a great many animals. Now a broader view of the economy of such tissue activity opens, and it surely will not fail to influence conceptions of health and disease.

But it is more than doubtful whether a new conception of the nature of disease and of the basis of general pathology will arise from this view. Disease will always have to be considered an altered vital state of larger or smaller numbers of cells or cell-territories, and, whether the cause of the disease circulates in the blood or arrives directly at the cells, our evaluation of the relationship of the primary causes to the cells will not change. Even immunization must in the last instance be related to living cells, regardless of where they are to be found. Science will surely discover the means to solve this problem.

Thus we see ourselves now at the conclusion of a century of hard work, not at the goal, but amidst a constantly increasing group of eager workers and in possession of new and highly improved methods and tools for investigation. Our understanding of disease is in accordance with the strictest demands of exact scientific investigation, and if the possibility of its interruption from time to time by arbitrary interpretations and speculative reveries has not been excluded, yet our science has become strong enough to follow the path unerringly in spite of all hindrances. May the coming century not stumble on this path! May a later generation, even after another one hundred years, still hold the banner of natural-scientific investigation as high as it is now held! Though that time may see advances still greater than those on which we labored together, yet no one will deny this expiring century a significant place in the history of medicine, a place more significant than that achieved by any earlier century.

The Berlin Pathological Institute can be regarded as an indicator of official esteem. From what was fifty years ago nothing more than the "morgue of the Charité," with extremely modest facilities, the Pathological Institute became in 1856, after the very incomplete attempt I made in Würzburg, the first great independent pathological institute in the world. In spite of considerable enlargement and improvement in 1876 and thereafter, we face once again the necessity of rebuilding in order to satisfy the greatly increased demands of instruction and investigation. In the course of a few decades every German university had added a pathological institute, and foreign countries are gradually beginning to follow this example. Simultaneously, numerous clinical institutes have been provided with scientific laboratories. Thus the new century begins with the confident hope that the path of independent pathological investigation is permanently secure.

Recent Progress in Science and Its Influence on Medicine and Surgery

(1898)

THE HONOR OF BEING INVITED to deliver the second of the Huxley Lectures has moved me deeply. How admirable are these days of commemoration, a national custom of the English people, whereby the memory of the spirit of heroes is kept alive for posterity! How affecting is this act of gratitude when such a celebration is held at the very place where the genius of the man it honors was first guided toward its scientific development! We are filled not only with admiration for the man, but also with appreciation for the institution which planted the seed of achievement in the soul of the young student.

That you, gentlemen, should have entrusted to a stranger the task of expressing these feelings seemed to me an act of such kindly sentiment, of such perfect confidence, that I at first hesitated to accept it. How am I to find in a strange tongue words which perfectly express my feelings? How can I, before a group of people unknown to me, many of whom knew this man and saw him at work, always find the right expression for what I wish to say as well as a member of that group could? I hesitate to believe that I shall be successful throughout. But if in spite of all I suppress my hesitation it is because I know how indulgent my English colleagues will be toward my often incomplete statements, and how much they are inclined to pardon deficiencies in diction when they are convinced of the good intentions of the speaker. I may assume that such a task would not have been allotted to me had not those who imposed it known how deeply the feeling of admiration for Huxley is rooted within me, had they not seen how fully I recognized the achievements of the departed master from the time of his first epoch-making publications, and how greatly I prized the friendship which he shared with me. In truth, the lessons that I received from him in his laboratory—a very modest one according to present standards—and the introduction to his work which I owe to him, form one of the most pleasant and lasting recollections of my visit to Kensington.

The most competent witness of Huxley's earliest period of development, Professor Foster, presented in the first of these lectures a picture of the rapidly moving progress of our biological knowledge, a picture which must have excited not only the admiration but the emulation of the younger generation of doctors and students. The task has been given me of incorporating in this picture the recent progress in science and its influence on medicine. So great is this task that it would be presumptuous even to attempt to accomplish it in a single lecture. I intend, therefore, to confine myself to a mere outline of the influence of the progress of biology on medicine. In this way also Huxley's career will become more intelligible to us.

Huxley himself, though trained in the practical school of Charing Cross Hospital, won his special title to fame in the field of biology. As a matter of fact, at that time the name "biology" had not yet come into general use. It is only in recent times, as I pointed out in my lecture "On the Place of Pathology Among the Biological Sciences," that the idea of life has received its full significance. Even in the late Middle Ages it lacked sufficient strength to struggle through the haze of dogmatism into the light. Today, for the second time, I am glad to give credit to the English nation for having made the first attempt to define the nature and characteristics of life. As I then pointed out, it was Francis Glisson who, following expressly in the footsteps of Paracelsus, discussed the *principium vitae*. If he could not elucidate the nature of life, he at least recognized its main characteristic. This is what he was the first to describe as "irritability," the characteristic on which the activity of living matter depends. He thus succeeded in setting aside the mystical idea of the spiritualistic *archaeus* which Paracelsus and his followers had placed in the foreground of discussion, and in locating the *principium energeticum* in matter itself.

What a step from Paracelsus to Glisson, and—we may add— from Glisson to Hunter! According to Paracelsus, life was the work of a special *spiritus* which set material substance in action, like a machine; for Glisson material substance was itself the *principium energeticum*. Unfortunately, he did not confine this dictum to living substances only, but applied it to substance in general, to all matter. It was Hunter who first emphasized the specific nature of living matter in contrast to non-living. But he too did not attain perfect clarity of vision, for in the development of English medicine the idea that life was not bound up with structure had been allowed to germinate and grow, so Hunter also was led to place a *materia vitae diffusa* at the head of his physiological and pathological ideas. Hence he arrived at the assumption of the so-called plastic substances, with the blood as mid-point and seat of origin. Thus it came about that in place of the old Greek humoral pathology, which Paracelsus had overthrown, a new humoral pathology arose—hematology. According to the teaching of Hewson and Hunter, the blood supplied the plastic materials of physiology as well as the plastic exudates of pathology.

Such was the basis of the new discipline of biology, if one can apply such an expression to an incomplete doctrine, when Huxley began his medical studies at Charing Cross Hospital in 1842. John Hunter was the accepted master of English pathology, and remained so for decades. So great was his influence that continental medicine recognized it as well. To this I can myself testify, as I was at that time finishing my university studies. It would lead us too far afield were I to depict at this point how it came about that, like Huxley, I too was early led away from the pernicious path of humoral pathology; suffice it to say that salvation came from the same science which had once before, in the sixteenth century, brought liberation from humoral pathology. This happened when Vesalius overthrew the authority of Galen and founded human anatomy upon direct observation, on necropsy. Since then anatomical instruction had been much widened and improved. When Huxley himself left Charing Cross Hospital in 1846, he had enjoyed an abundance of instruction in anatomy and physiology. How great this was can be gathered from the interesting statistics which Professor Foster has collected with the aid of Huxley's distinguished fellow student, Sir Joseph Fayrer. Of the lectures which junior students attended, one hundred and forty in each of the three years of study were devoted to anatomy and physiology. Thus prepared, Huxley took the post of naval surgeon, and by the time he returned, four years later, he had become an accomplished zoologist and an acute ethnologist.

How this was possible will be readily understood by anyone who knows from his own experience how great is the value of personal observation for the development of independent and unprejudiced thought. For a young man who, besides collecting a rich store of positive knowledge, has practiced dissection and exercised critical judgment, a long sea voyage and a peaceful sojourn among entirely new surroundings afford an invaluable opportunity for original work and deep reflection. Freed from the formalism of the schools, thrown upon the use of his own intellect, compelled to test each object with respect to its properties and history, he soon forgets the dogmas of the prevailing system and becomes first a skeptic and then an investigator. This change, acting upon Huxley, out of which came the Huxley whom we commemorate today, is not an unknown occurrence to one who is acquainted with the history of individual scholars, as well as the history of knowledge. We need only point to John Hunter and Darwin as related examples.

The path on which these men achieved their triumphs is that on which biology as a whole has trodden with ever-lengthening strides since the end of the previous century; it is the path of genetic investigation. We Germans point with pride to our fellow countryman who opened up this road with full conviction of its importance and who turned the eyes of the world toward it—our poet-prince Goethe. What he accomplished for plants, others of our countrymen did for animals. I recall Caspar Friedrich Wolff, Döllinger, Johann Friedrich Meckel, Carl von Baer, and our whole embryological school. As Harvey, Haller, and Hunter had done, these men began with the study of the "ovulum," but it soon became plain that the egg itself was organized, and that from it arose the whole series of organic developments. When Huxley, after his return, published his fundamental observations, he found the natural history of the progressive transformations of the contents of the egg already verified, for it was now known that the egg was a cell, and that from it other cells and, in turn, the organs arose. The second of his three famous papers, on the relationship between man and the nearest related animals, sketched in masterful fashion the parallelism found in the earliest development of all animals. More than this it stepped boldly across the borderline which tradition and dogma had drawn between man and the animals. Huxley had no hesitation in filling the gap which Darwin had left in his argument, and in stating "that in respect to substance and structure man and the lower animals are one."

Whatever opinion one may hold about the origin of man, the fundamental correspondence of human organization with that of animals is at present universally accepted. From this correspondence all biological disciplines, especially physiology and pathology, derive the urge to comparative studies. In particular, all that is to be based on experiment must first be investigated in animals. All that requires morphological confirmation finds support in comparative anatomy, histology, and embryology. The basis of our current theory of medicine actually rests on finer microscopy, for whose elaboration animal tissues form an indispensable control. Suffice it to say that in scientific biology the division between man and animal becomes less and less clear, but only, let it be noted, the division between abstract man and abstract animal. It is the same situation that we meet in differentiating between plants and animals. How many definitions of this have been put forth in the course of time, and how many, one after the other, have collapsed! But if we place a specific animal and a specific plant side by side we overcome the difficulties which we ourselves create with our definitions.

The greatest difficulty in biology has arisen because man, following a natural tendency, has put the search for the unitary basis of life in the foreground of his attention. As a matter of fact, what is more natural than the conclusion that life as a special phenomenon must also have a special basis, and that the material process of life must be derived from a common cause? During the last century an attempt was made to satisfy this claim by the assumption, made with continually increasing conviction, of a special force—the life-force. Today we can see the logical errors which permitted this assumption. Time has, however, passed its judgment, and today no one continues to speak of vital force. And yet the necessity for a single basis of all vital manifestations remains. How is this to be satisfied? This is a question which not only is of great theoretical interest, but has led to the construction of a foundation indispensable for practical work, and particularly for medical practice. But in order to reach this foundation, it is first of all necessary to dispense with all the dogmas of the schools, and to seek an objective picture of the nature of vital processes.

Man, the higher animals, and plants, as regards material construction, are not unitary beings; on the contrary, they are put together from many separate units. Hence they are called organisms. If a single force which set all their parts in action was within them, it would be impossible to conceive the origin of the special kind of activity exhibited by each of these organisms in its own special fashion. This specific activity is present in the organism not only in its final or fully developed form, but also during development and growth. How could a single force, whether we call it, in the spiritualistic sense, spirit, soul, *spiritus rector*, or, in the physical sense, vital force or electricity, build up such diverse organisms? Or if this force resided in a single organ —whether in brain, spinal cord, or heart—how could we explain those creatures without brains or hearts, which seem so abnormal that at the beginning of this century their condition was the play-ground of the mystics?

In my opinion, there is only one solution possible. The life possessed by the higher organisms is not unitary. Their life and all their activities become intelligible only when we go back to the exact conception, based upon a kind of intuitive observation, of the life of their individual parts. Each constituent part of a living organism has its special life, its *vita propria*. None of the older authors proclaimed this more distinctly than Paracelsus. But he at once spoiled this good idea by attributing to each living part a particular *spiritus*, a special *archaeus*. The best of the suc-ceeding biologists were also caught by this notion as by a snare; instead of busying themselves with observation of the *vita propria* —that is, the activity of the individual parts—they continued to seek for the *archaeus*.

The advances in general science based on dissection, particu-larly those in medicine, have completely turned the attention of true investigators to the study of individual parts. As I pointed out at the Medical Congress at Rome,[1] the history of pathology clearly shows that it was the division of the body first into larger regions (head, breast, abdomen, etc.), then into organs, tissues, and finally into cells and cell territories, which gave us under-standing of disease. The study of regions was followed by the study of organs, by the study of the tissues, and finally by the cell theory. What is true of pathology holds also for physiology, and indeed physiology has passed through the same stages of development. One gradually comes to understand that the life of the individual part is fully comprehensible if we forget about the *archaei* of the organs and tissues, and keep in mind the life and activities of single cells. For the life of an organ is nothing other than the sum of the lives of the single cells gathered to-gether into it, and the life of the whole organism is not an indi-vidual but a collective activity.

If such a collective being is to be analyzed, no matter whether the whole organism, a single organ, or a single tissue displays its vital activity, the first requisite for a correct interpretation is that one should discard its fancied unity, and regard the single parts, the cells, as the bearers of life. Single cells can be separated out even in a complex organism. We should with some difficulty arrive at a satisfactory theory if we did not also find single free-living cells in nature. These have provided the basis for objective investigation. During this century unicellular plants and animals have been more frequently and adequately studied. Botanists and zoologists have become the teachers of physiologists and pathologists. The ova of animals and the corresponding germ cells of plants have bridged the gap between single free-living cells and the higher organisms. It was the recognition of this fact which first raised the famous dictum of Harvey to the high position which it merits.

In a medical school, where the teaching is almost entirely concerned with human beings, we might put this sentence at the head of the lesson: *The organism is not a single unit, but a social system*. An exact anatomical analysis of this system always brings us finally to cells; they are the ultimate constituents and the origin of all tissues. Hence we call them the living elements and regard them as the anatomical basis of all biological analysis, whether it has a physiological or pathological object in view.

In this connection two assumptions must be made: (1) every organism, like every organ and tissue, contains cells as long as it is alive; (2) the cells are composed of organic chemical substances, themselves not alive, whose mechanical arrangement determines the direction and power of their activity.

The first proposition has slowly been accepted in recent years. Schwann, who recognized the origin of tissues from cells, still clung to the opinion that in the further development of many tissues the cells disappeared. Among these he reckoned the important class which has subsequently been called the connective tissues because they maintain the form and stability of single organs, and of the whole organism. First among these are the osseous and connective tissues, which form a large part of the tissue make-up of the higher organisms. The notion that the osseous and connective tissues are free from cells must now be given up. Where formerly only empty spaces or gaps (*lacunae*) were seen in the tissues, we can now demonstrate cells. We can even isolate them. Hence it is now desirable that the name "tissue," in the sense of living tissue, should be applied only to parts that contain living cells. In addition to the cells the tissue may contain a more or less abundant quantity of organic (chemical) material, but this intercellular or extracellular substance must be regarded as a product rather than a carrier of life. Parts which arose originally from living cells, but whose cells have perished, must be excluded from biological consideration. As examples may be adduced the epidermis, the hair, and the enamel of the teeth. These consist in reality of dead tissue.

With regard to the second proposition, that no organic chemical substance is alive, it has been objected that all living matter is put together from organic chemical materials. Those who raise this objection overlook the fact that these two kinds of substance, living and non-living, cannot be identified. In spite of chemical similarity or even correspondence, they exhibit recognizable differences, not alone physiological, but also mechanical and physical. Since the use of dyes has given us a glimpse of the variety of the finer mechanical, or one may say molecular, arrangements of matter, it has become possible to differentiate living and non-living parts *de visu*. We are admittedly only on the threshold of these investigations, but the most recent investigations of ganglion cells have shown that, in addition to differences in staining, living and dead parts may be optically distinguishable otherwise.

The enthusiasm with which for centuries the doctrine of formative principles and nutritive materials was built up has already abated, and the doctrine has in part been entirely abandoned, owing to the knowledge that no single chemical substance, no kind of nutritive or formative material which can be immediately employed as such for the production or formation of cells, has ever been found outside the living organism. And yet a chemist of Liebig's importance actually believed that fibrin could be conveyed directly from ingested meat into the fluids of the body, and thence into the tissues. This was based on a misconception— a relic from the time of the old humoral pathology—the living body and its constituent parts being regarded as the product of a combination of a few basic substances (*humores cardinales*).

Thus originated the doctrine of plastic materials, which were supposed to be preexistent in the food and blood. With obstinacy only surpassed by their superficiality these theorists remained convinced that the plastic materials as such effected the construction and maintenance of living matter. They failed to see that the nutriment taken in had first to be prepared by special juices secreted by cells of the digestive organs, and that both the digestive material and the plastic substance of the blood were rendered assimilable by means of a new change, effected by the agency of tissue cells.

The doctrine of plastic material appeared to have gained new strength with Schwann's cell theory. One must be careful not to misunderstand his theory. Since the cell theory of animal and plant life has been confirmed, many have maintained that Schwann's theory is identical with it. Not only is this not the case, but the two stand in exact opposition to one another. Schwann assumed, and believed, that he had directly observed the origin of cells from undifferentiated matter, from a fluid or semi-solid mass, in the following way: first small firm particles separated off, and then they came together into little clumps and masses which gradually changed into cell nuclei. A new precipitate of firmer substance now slowly accumulated around this, and the body of the cell appeared. Hence the original amorphous substance would be the actual formative material, while the cell was formed by the nucleus; Schwann called the former the cytoblastema, the latter the cytoblast.

It is obvious that such a premise logically led to the conclusion that every form of organic tissue or organism, every formation of new cells, must be separated from the preceding by a definite gap (*hiatus*), and that each new formation must be considered a discontinuous vital process. Strangely enough, this classification arose and was accepted at a time when Darwin was already at work proving that new species arise by the modification of preexisting forms. But Schwann's cell theory was in truth a resuscitation of the archaic doctrine of spontaneous generation (*generatio aequivoca, epigenesis*). Darwinism was incompatible with the domination of such a creed.

The supports of *generatio aequivoca* have been, as far as zoology is concerned, gradually demolished. The formation of tissue cells from the cleavage of the ovum has been observed throughout the whole animal kingdom. Animals apparently without ova, such as the cestoids and trichinae, have successively been brought under Harvey's law; we are acquainted with their ova, their embryos, and their path through the tissues. There remained finally but one domain, though this was large and of the highest importance, belonging particularly to pathology. It was that of the plastic exudates, which accompany the most important clinical processes, in particular the inflammatory process.

It will readily be understood why a subject so proper to pathology should have had little interest for pure natural scientists. They left it to medical men, who are occupied with it every day. But in medicine this domain was held sacrosanct; no one doubted that old, well-attested experience spoke here. We older physicians were brought up in this belief; we mastered the doctrine of the so-called plastic exudates in our earliest studies. Translated into our current parlance, this doctrine would recognize discontinuity in the majority of pathological new formations; it would establish—and this is worth noting—a basis for the dogma of the origin of life from non-living matter. Experience, however, has taught us that exactly the opposite is true.

Permit me here, gentlemen, to speak from a more personal standpoint than I shall elsewhere. It will, perhaps, be more understandable for the students at this school, and make more of an impression, if I tell how I myself arrived at quite different views.

It was toward the end of my academic studies, more than fifty years ago, that I began work as an assistant in the ophthalmic clinic of the Charité Hospital at Berlin. My attention was at once drawn to diseases of the cornea. We had cases of severe keratitis, but I observed no exudation here. Numerous operations for cataract were performed and wounds closed, without the formation of plastic exudates; they were not seen in corneal scars. Could this be explained by the fact that the cornea, except at its periphery, is an avascular tissue? My interest was at once focused on such avascular tissues. I turned first to the articular cartilages, and here also I found great changes in the absence of exudation, certainly of plastic exudation. I need only recall the form of inflammation which I named *arthritis chronica deformans*, and which is described by French physicians as *arthrite sèche*. My experimental studies on the inflammation of blood vessels showed that the intima, likewise avascular, of the larger arteries, and in part also that of the veins, can undergo great changes without even a trace of exudation. Later anatomical investigations on endocarditis led to the same result, provided that parietal thrombi are not regarded as exudates. But everywhere and in every instance there were changes in the tissue cells, active changes such as swelling, multiplication of nuclei, etc., or passive changes such as fatty degeneration.

Next I turned to vascular organs, and in particular to those which were recognized as the common sites of exudative processes. I refer, first, to the medullary infiltration of the lymphatic (follicular) tissue of the intestine and the mesenteric glands seen in typhoid fever, and so strikingly depicted by the Vienna school. Instead of the amorphous albuminous exudate which was described, I found cells, cells of the same kind as those normally present. Likewise in the so-called caseous exudates which were at one time ascribed to scrofula, at another to tuberculosis; the cheesy material was admittedly for the most part amorphous, but it was actually not an exudate at all, not a primary product of disease but rather a secondary product of degenerative, necrobiotic changes in tissues which had formerly been organized and not infrequently actually hyperplastic.

It is not necessary to go into further details in order to show the magnitude of the realm of pseudo-exudative processes. But I must refer to another group of morbid processes affecting the bones. It was while studying rickets that I first recognized the biological significance of the cartilage corpuscles, which had till then been interpreted in a variety of ways. I believe that I was the first to distinguish in these corpuscles the cells from the merely capsular and extracellular coverings. The rachitic disturbance clearly demonstrated a phenomenon that was repeatedly misunderstood, even by later observers: the increase of these cells by division, and the consequent growth of the cartilage.

It was not difficult to follow the direct transition of epiphysial cartilage into the periosteum of the neighboring bone, thus into connective tissue. At this time the whole world was convinced of the correctness of Duhamel's statement that increase in thickness of the long bones was effected by the exudation of a nutritious fluid from the periosteal vessels, out of which new bone substance was formed. Pathologists had extended this to cover periostitis and the formation of exostoses and hyperostoses; they supposed that between the periosteum and the bone a plastic exudation was secreted and stored up, and that the osteophytes arose by secondary organization. The results of my studies showed that in none of these sites, neither in cartilage nor in periosteum, was cellular organization in normal growth, rickets, or periostitis preceded by the appearance of a recognizable amorphous exudate. On the contrary, it was clearly evident that the first stage was an active, productive process of cell multiplication, while at the same time the intercellular substance altered in character and underwent a series of changes until it took on the appearance of osteoid; not until then did calcification and true ossification occur. There was no difficulty in adducing proof that the separate stages of these processes ran a parallel course in cartilage and in periosteum, although the new tissue was in the one case true cartilage, in the other only cartilage-like. If one wishes to give a name to this general process, it ought to be called proliferation. Whoever believes that the proliferative layer is an exudate will never obtain an objective understanding of the actual course of events.

There is thus not the slightest necessity for a true observer to retain the arbitrary and totally erroneous notion of plastic exudation. There is no such thing as a simple amorphous plastic exudate; the cells found in it did not originate from it. With this demonstration, which can be shown in numerous other instances, the idea of the discontinuous origin of pathological new formations must be discarded. Every new tissue formation presupposes a tissue from which its cells arise; this tissue is its matrix.

There is no difference in principle between the descent of men and animals from one parent and the descent of pathological new formations from one matrix. Pathology has been somewhat late in arriving at an understanding of this correspondence, but I think it has particular value for all fields of biology.

In order to avoid a misunderstanding, it should be noted that not every living cell is capable of becoming a matrix. All cells destined for the highest animal functions prove sterile, or at least capable of only limited proliferation. Ganglion cells, primitive muscle bundles, and red blood corpuscles are not to be included in the theory of pathological descent. More indifferent cells, on the other hand, in particular those of cartilage, connective tissue, and epithelium, exhibit a striking ability to bring forth new cells. Many cells such as bone corpuscles and fat cells require a special preparatory metaplastic stage before they can produce new descendants.

Proliferation is thus a property of special cells. That it is not common to all cells alike in no way alters the fact that it can be performed only by cells. Just as little is it a function of an entire organism, for such an organism would itself have to be unicellular. In this property lies the explanation of the origin of whole organisms from single ova, that wonderful process which happens but once in the life of an organism. Once tissues have been formed, each cell of a tissue matrix may in respect to proliferation be compared to an ovum; it brings forth a new progeny from which new tissue is formed. This tissue bears, as a rule, the stamp of its matrix—it is modeled after the parental type. This is the nature of descent, and herein lies the key to an understanding of heredity, that puzzling phenomenon which has concerned mankind for so long.

According to the humoral theory heredity was rooted in the fluids of the body, in particular in the blood. According to this idea the blood was the source of propagation of the family and the race; blood relationship explained the similarity not only of the fluids but also of the organs and of the whole body. According to its nature, the blood determined the goodness or badness of the organism; noble blood generated noblemen and healthy organs, bad blood a debased posterity and organs predisposed to disease. In scientific work nothing remains of these fantastic surmises; they persist like a superstition in lay circles, but no one now seriously maintains their correctness. In their place has arisen a recognition of the particular importance of the parent tissue and its cells. These are the bearers of inherited characteristics, the sources of the germs of new tissues, and the engines of vital activity.

During the development of higher organisms the constitution of the individual tissues changes; they become differentiated by means of metaplastic processes connected with cells and cell territories. Thus it comes about that people have, since antiquity, spoken of *dissimilar* parts. The complete and fully developed organism is built up of similar and dissimilar tissues; their harmonious working together gives the impression of a unity of the whole organism which is actually nonexistent. For the more the organism develops, the more its social character becomes evident. It consists of innumerable independent parts which together form a single social body. If we wish to designate the ultimate elements of these parts, we must call them cells, without exception, for cells alone are truly alive, and scientific judgment is in the last analysis concerned with them.

The whole organism is so little a definite unit that the number of its living constituents is highly variable. Looking at the gross arrangement of the organs, we become accustomed to regard a certain number of them as typical of human beings and of the various genera and species of animals. We expect to find two of the paired organs, and one of the unpaired, in a single individual. Man, like all other animals, has a fixed number of bones and teeth, and these numbers are rightly used to characterize man or particular varieties and species of animal. But these numbers form no essential feature of existence; a man with six fingers or seven toes remains a man, just as a lung with supernumerary lobes or a kidney with an excess of medullary pyramids (*coni medullares*) remains a lung or a kidney. A woman with three, four, or even more mammary glands is no more a lower animal than a man with a tail. These are anomalies (theromorphs) which have no influence on our judgment of the sex or position in the animal scale of the affected individual.

But it will be a long time before general opinion on the significance of such anomalies will, even among experts, become unanimous. One group will relate them to descent, and find in them a proof of atavism, while another will regard them only as pathological formations, and will trace them back to acquired lesions. During the last century there have been violent disputes over whether certain malformations were inherited or acquired. Those who declared themselves for inheritance generally had the additional idea that the variation was atavistic. If they were acquainted with the entire animal kingdom, they cared little whether the atavism was derivable from human ancestors, or whether one would have to go back as far as the lower animals to account for it. A universally valid explanation of theromorphism has not yet been found. In my opinion it will never be found. Each single example must be separately studied and explained, and the general value of the explanation will be by no means established if we find atavism in a single case. Doubtless an acquired variation can also be transmitted, and the circumstance that it is animal-like (theroid) does not prove that it is atavistic, rather than the result of inherited transmission. In connection with this I may refer to my paper on race formation and heredity.[2] I can here discuss only the chief basis of the disputes regarding hereditary diseases in the field of pathology.

Medical men are accustomed to describe as hereditary all diseases which reappear in different generations of the same family. Thus they speak of hereditary arthritis, hereditary tuberculosis, and hereditary cancer. It is in fact not difficult to produce genealogical tables which demonstrate the recurrence of a paternal or a maternal disease in the children or grandchildren. Much effort has been devoted, in my opinion without result, to seeking the germs of such diseases in the ovum or the sperm cell. One is compelled to move on to generations of cells originating after conception. Here we reach what Roux[3] has designated the post-generative formations. The further we pass from the time of conception, the more numerous the examples of alterations in the formation of cells and embryonic tissues. But the possibility becomes more likely that the disturbance arose after the formation of the first cells, and hence that the cause began to act at that time. If we set aside this possibility, nothing else remains but to assume that at the time of conception, or even from the organs which produced the ovum or the spermatozoon, a predisposition (*Anlage*) is transmitted which is already present in the earliest cells, even though it cannot be detected.

Upon this theory are based all interpretations of the inheritance of pathological and, we may add, physiological structures. There are, for example, many extraordinary anomalies in the disposition of hair—excesses and defects—and nothing is more common than to observe hereditary transmission of such anomalies. But hairs are postgenerative structures, and a disturbance in their development can make its first appearance only in a late period of fetal life; not infrequently, indeed, such disturbances are first seen after birth. If such a peculiarity appears in many generations of a family or a race, it is called hereditary and referred to as a hereditary predisposition. But since excesses as well as defects in hair formation undoubtedly occur in acquired disturbances, in actual diseases, it becomes necessary to find causes for such anomalies as well. If one is found, a predisposition need not, as a rule, be invoked; one may rest contented with the cause, the *causa efficiens*.

Recent medical history affords a most striking example of a rapid and far-reaching change in the interpretation of a disease formerly regarded as hereditary. Leprosy was for thousands of years regarded as contagious. But about a generation ago, when the number of lepers in Norway increased to an astounding extent and one family after another was seized by the malady, the question of its hereditary character arose. Zealous investigators ransacked genealogical tables and church registers, and families were discovered in which leprosy had persisted for decades, even centuries. So universal was this conviction that the government, with the consent of the clergy, wished to promulgate a decree forbidding marriage in such cases; only by a small majority in Parliament was the proposal rejected. I was then requested by the government to travel through the leprous districts and to make a report; I succeeded in collecting a small number of verified cases in which all suspicion of heredity could be excluded. These were patients who came as healthy adults from regions free of leprosy into the infected districts, and after a long sojourn there developed leprosy.

A few years later Armauer Hansen[4] discovered the leprosy bacillus. Medical opinion changed in a moment. The ancient idea of the contagiousness of the disease was revived. Inheritance was denied and predisposition vanished from the store of dogmas. I will not assert that the grounds for embracing the present view are absolutely convincing, but I am positive that this view is much to be preferred to the dogma of heredity. It should be instructive to all of us that one single fact, the discovery of a *causa viva*, sufficed to overthrow an apparently well-based theory. Well-established knowledge of a cause has at once converted leprosy from an inherited into an acquired disease.

A similar thing happened a few decades earlier with two skin diseases which, according to the views of humoral pathology, were traceable to a change in the blood, to a dyscrasia, namely tinea (favus, porrigo) and scabies (the "itch"). The first actually bore the name of *tinea hereditaria*, and in German was called *Erbgrind*. But the microscope revealed to Schönlein that tinea was caused by a mycelial fungus. With regard to scabies the view of Italian folk medicine, that a mite (*Acarus*) caused it, was confirmed. So unstable are the most plausible theories in the light of objective, factual knowledge.

Experience has been the same in connection with certain diseases of the hair. When fungi were found on the hairs, no one troubled further about predisposition, although this possibly does occur. While it is certain that there are parasitic forms of alopecia, fungi cannot be found in every instance. Still less is this the case in anomalies of the hair characterized by excessive growth. Here no other explanation than the assumption of a predisposition is possible. This holds equally for hirsute races and for families of men with excessive hair, as well as for those single hairy cutaneous patches (*naevi pilosi*) which are regarded as hereditary. The hair roots carry the predisposition, those which arise during fetal life and thus belong to the postgenerative group, but which do not show increased activity until much later.

The general cutaneous covering, in brief the skin, although doubtless a kind of unitary structure showing general similarity, is nevertheless in a double sense a socially constituted organ. Not only is it composed of numerous independent cells and cell territories of different kinds—apart from the vessels and nerves—the connective tissue, the cutis proper, and the horny epithelial tissue which forms hairs and glands, but also the individual constituents of the skin have special predispositions and are exposed to various external and internal influences. This is best shown by the numerous morbid states to whose scientific classification the English dermatologists so early devoted themselves. The existence of macular, papular, pustular, and all the various other kinds of skin eruptions is made possible because in the skin a number of little communities appear from the beginning as independent, hereditary, bearers of particular predispositions. When birthmarks (*naevi*), hairs, or even spines arise from these foci, it follows that in spite of their common origin there must be lasting differences between them.

There is another highly remarkable question which every year increases its claim on the attention of medical men. This was formerly described as *aberratio loci*, and is now called *heterotopia*. It has long been known that hairs occur not only on the skin, where they properly belong, but also in internal organs, where they are quite out of place; and further, that other cutaneous structures such as epidermis, sebaceous glands, and cutis may be present as well. We group these under the general term "dermoid." Modern histologists have long struggled against the hypothesis of aberration, but they have finally had to surrender, and the view has become dominant that in fetal life smaller or larger rudimentary fragments can indeed separate from their natural abodes and move to other loci, where they find a new home, so to speak, and can undergo all the further changes proper to their cutaneous origin. Cysts and other tumors can thus arise.

The most remarkable examples of such heterotopias are afforded by certain glandular organs which under normal conditions appear as communities composed of similar parts, arranged in characteristic order. Among them an important place is occupied by two organs, the thyroid gland and the adrenal glands, which have recently demanded much attention. On their surfaces the pushing forward and progressive isolation of separate parts, in the form of nodules or small lobes, can be observed. But occasionally these nodules leave the main body of the gland and are found completely detached in quite unusual sites more or less removed from their seat of origin. The broken-off nodules of the suprarenals are more widely distributed; their wanderings lead them to adjacent zones on the kidneys, or even into the interior of the kidneys, and in other instances beyond the kidneys into the peritoneum as far down as the pelvic basin. And in all these places they may undergo further changes, and even become starting points of tumors.

The same aberration has long been recognized in teeth, and it is known that large tumors can arise from heterotopic tooth germs. The same is true of cartilage, where similar displacements occur in fetal life. The natural history of rickets has shown us that islands of cartilage originally connected with the primary cartilages of the epiphyses or diaphyses later come, in the course of bone growth, to be completely separated from their matrix. New formations such as enchondromata and osseous cysts may thus arise.

Extraordinary, even astonishing, as many of these instances are, they lose the strangeness which they show on superficial examination if we recall a common kind of heterotopia, first used among the people and then in surgical practice, and finally studied experimentally as "transplantation." Since the grafting of pieces of the epidermis has come into use in rhinoplasty, and has often been applied with great success in the treatment of refractory ulcers, it is no longer surprising to think that living tissue may survive and undergo further development in unwonted situations. Experimentally and in surgical practice first place is taken by the transplantation of periosteum, which can be carried into every possible corner of the body, even through the circulation into the lungs, conserving in all of these places its vitality and its power of serving as a matrix for osseous tissue.

In my opinion, the theoretical significance of these observations has been exaggerated in so far as a property possessed by the transplanted tissue, the property of forming a tumor by proliferation, has been made the explanation of tumor formation in general. This is a mistake. Transplanted tissue has no fresh properties beyond those of the mother tissue in which it arises.

That a sarcoma can arise from a nevus is only possible because the latter is a part of the skin, and because the skin itself can also produce sarcomata. A cartilaginous tumor can arise from aberrant pieces of cartilage in the middle of a bone, and give rise to an enchondroma, but one may also arise from permanent cartilage in the form of an outgrowth (ecchondrosis). A dermoid cyst can serve as a site of origin of a cutaneous horn, but cutaneous horns and spines also grow from ordinary skin. In each of these instances there is only the possibility of formation present in the parent tissue. At the same time each of these instances illustrates the law of the *vita propria* of the parts, and of their corresponding activity.

It is not without great scientific and practical interest to reflect that these observations illustrate another ancient doctrine, that of parasitism. This doctrine, too, is traceable back to Paracelsus and his wish to have disease in general regarded as a parasite. One century after another has transmitted this theory, or at least kept its memory green, although there is a fundamental error of logic in assuming the universality of parasitism. Not every disease is parasitic. If this were the case, we should have to regard the life of the whole organism as parasitic. For if the living organism is constituted by separate and independent living parts, each of which nourishes itself, and most of which can propagate themselves and perform their special functions, each one of these individual parts is a parasite with respect to the others; it lives on and lessens the common stock of nourishment. The generally accepted view regarding parasitism postulates at the same time its harmful character. In reality, every part is endowed with individual life in such a manner that it can harm the remainder of the organism if its activity becomes excessive or defective. A nevus that becomes a sarcoma is extremely dangerous. Hence it is requisite to remove a sarcoma, but it is not advisable to remove every nevus. Only an excess of caution can lead to an operation which finds its sole excuse in the possibility that a nevus can lead to the formation of a sarcoma. In like manner every excessive proliferation can be harmful; it may then be described as malignant. But many proliferative processes are benign or even useful, as, for instance, the scar tissue which replaces defects. It is for the sake of a trustworthy prognosis that one must be extremely careful in grouping whole categories of morbid processes under a common name.

The idea of parasitism, which we have here discussed in regard to the relation between different parts of the same organism, is more applicable where living organisms of a different variety or species enter into an organism and continue their special life within it. The animal parasites, which live as entozoa in man and other animals, have been longest known. Since the end of the last century our acquaintance with these entozoa has greatly broadened. Many structures which were formerly regarded as mere cysts have been recognized as cestoid worms (*entozoa cystica*). The trichinae, apparently sexless animals living in the interior of muscles, were first discovered in this century at Edinburgh; later experimental research proved that after the consumption of infected meat these tiny worms rapidly become sexually ripe in the bowel and produce living embryos and larvae, as well as ova. Then there are the worms which live in the blood, the distomata and filariae, and later wander into the tissues. All have a period during which they dwell as organozoa in the midst of the living tissues of the host organism, and become so perfectly incorporated that they carry on their own lives just like the proper cells.

Quite new, and exclusively a development of investigation in our own time, are the parasitic protozoa, beings of so rudimentary a kind that their position in the biological system is even yet not quite clear. Chief among these are the malarial protozoa, microscopic organisms, many of which are so tiny that they can penetrate into the smallest cells, such as the red blood corpuscles. The darkness which for thousands of years enveloped a group of highly dangerous diseases—the tropical fevers—has been dispelled by the discovery of these tiny creatures. Important stages in the natural history of these parasites are still unknown; we know nothing definite about their origin or occurrence outside the great organisms which are their temporary dwelling places, and nothing, also, about their mode of action within these organisms, but we hold the threads by means of which complete knowledge will be attained.

Lastly comes the equally new field of microscopic plants which appear as mere grains (cocci), or as minute rods or chains (bacilli), and from which many of the most severe diseases, the elite of the parasitic infectious maladies, take origin. Their recognition began with the study of two very important and widespread processes, fermentation and putrefaction. It will remain the imperishable achievement of Pasteur that he firmly established the dependence of these processes on the activity of microbes, and that he elucidated their further life history, and their power of producing active chemical or physico-chemical substances. Here, for the first time, parasitic beings which live and carry on their work outside the organism were subjected to experimental study. Here were obtained the wonderful results which have opened new paths both in medicine and in technical science. The results of microscopic research have been supported everywhere by trustworthy experiments, and their significance has been established beyond all doubt. Pathology, in particular, has achieved, in fields which had hitherto eluded investigation, a degree of clarity and certainty which has been reached in few other disciplines.

The first great stride in the special domain of pathology was made in veterinary medicine. The discovery of the anthrax bacillus by Brannel disclosed the new group of pathogenic bacilli, as we now call them. It would lead us too far afield to refer to all of these, or even to enumerate them; it must suffice to mention the two worst diseases whose dreadful effects are due to the action of bacilli—tuberculosis and Asiatic cholera. In both cases it was Robert Koch who, with careful and often very delicate procedures, succeeded in demonstrating the invariable presence of specific bacilli in the tissues. It was seen that in spite of the presence of bacilli in both diseases a totally different kind of infection occurred in the two; while the tubercle bacilli invade the organs, and develop their deadly action in them, the cholera bacilli remain almost exclusively in the intestine and grow more after the manner of infusorial plants.

For our discussion today it is inadvisable to go into more minute details. Only a few of the more important points can be discussed. One of them I will mention only briefly, since I have written many lengthy papers on it: the necessity for distinguishing between the inciting cause (*causa*) and the essential nature (*essentia*) of infectious diseases. Parasitic beings, specifically bacteria, are never more than inciting causes; the nature of the disease depends upon the behavior of the organs or tissues affected by the bacteria or their metabolic products. In my opinion this distinction is of cardinal importance.

My other two points require somewhat fuller discussion. The first is the general relation of the smaller parasites to the diseases determined by them. Under one designation, "infection," which reaches back even into the old days of humoral pathology, and which I was the first to reintroduce into common parlance, are grouped together all the processes produced by the invasion of pathogenic substances. The Latin word *inficere* means "to pollute." The polluting substance (*res inficiens*) has been called for ages an "impurity" (*impuritas*). The products of putrefaction (*materiae putridae*) served as its prototype. In Greek they were called miasms (from μιαίνω, *inficio*), so that these names were applied chiefly to such polluting agents as were produced outside the body; those arising inside the human or animal body were called "contagions." Both miasmatic and contagious substances produced, after their penetration into the body, severe effects resembling poisoning. To distinguish such substances from true poisons (*venena*) they were designated "viruses." A relationship between infection and intoxication was recognized, but it was not without good reason, considering the origin of the impurities, that the difference in nomenclature was retained.

Among the innumerable infectious diseases it was the "contagions," since they endangered the health and life not only of individual men and animals but of large groups as well, which became most prominent. Notice was taken of their remarkable ability to multiply in the body and so to produce an immense quantity of fresh virulent substance, in addition to the infection as such. In this respect they resembled living beings, and the idea arose that they themselves were alive (*contagia viva*). With the discovery of parasitic animals and plants this conjecture was verified. Nothing was easier than to generalize from this and to expect the presence of independent organisms in every contagious disease. With fiery enthusiasm the younger generation of doctors and students disregarded the necessity of proof, and succumbed to the conviction that all infection depended on invasion by parasitic organisms. And since it was precisely the most severe infections which were produced by the minute plants, and since among these bacilli and cocci, or, as they are called, "bacteria," were most often found, that beatific axiom "Infection is pollution by bacteria" circulated for a considerable time.

It should have been known that parasitic animals and protozoa can also give rise to infection, and that between bacteria and fungi there is more than a slight difference, but for convenience the name "bacteria" was retained as a general designation. Further, there was the peculiar circumstance that there were no botanical names for most of the so-called bacteria. Owing to the novelty of the circumstances, botanists have even yet not succeeded, according to their usual custom, in giving every new kind its special name, in determining its genus and species, and in assigning it a place in a systematic classification. This can easily be understood and forgiven. But it does not in any way alter the fallacious character of a method which attributes every "impurity" to bacteria solely because of its contagiousness. It may be said that the contagious character of a disease suggests its bacterial origin, but it should not be regarded as bacterial forthwith. To do so hinders further research and dulls the conscience.

Some of the most important contagious diseases have resisted all attempts to find parasitic contagia in them. Many have been the hopes of finding the parasite of venereal disease, and just as many have been the failures. The coccus of gonorrhea alone has been discovered; the bacterium of syphilis itself remains a *pium desiderium*. With even more certainty it was expected that a pathological parasite would be found in variola; more than one bacterium was actually found, but none were pathogenic. All appearances seemed to promise that hydrophobia (*lyssa*, rabies) would prove to be a microparasitic disease. Its contagious character is indubitable, and a vaccine, as with smallpox, has even been prepared, yet no one has been able to culture a specific bacillus. And the same is the case with some of the most dreaded contagious diseases. Painful as it may be, one can do nothing but wait, observe, and experiment. Perhaps pathogenic bacteria will be found, but as long as they are not discovered all certainty is useless, if not actually dangerous. To have learned this is a good omen for our progress in scientific method.

The second point in the doctrine of infectious diseases, which has been the subject of much investigation, is the question of the mode of action of infectious agents. As long as infection by animal parasites was regarded as the prototype of infection in general, the destructive effect was considered to be the result of mechanical action, comparable to biting or devouring. But precise study of the larger entozoa soon blighted this hope. Neither taenia solium nor taenia echinococcus has an oral opening. They undoubtedly take in nourishment and draw it from their autosites —their "hosts," as they are fancifully called—but this applies only to the absorption of fluids. The intake of food by bacteria and other plant and plantlike parasites has to be regarded in more or less the same way. Certainly they injure the tissues and organs in which they reside by consuming important materials, but their activity is not limited to this effect. This much we have already learned in the study of fermentation and putrefaction. It is admitted that they destroy organic matter, but in addition they produce new substances, some of which are eminently poisonous. It has been known for centuries that alcohol is produced by fermentation. For a long time the putrefactive poisons could not be isolated; first Selmi and then Brieger succeeded in this. Gradually one ptomaine after the other has been found. The new term "toxin" has been introduced by Brieger in place of the old term "virus." They are chemical substances, in part crystallizable, or at least diffusible, linked neither with cells nor with other formed elements, though produced by cellular activity on the part of the parasites. They are today often described as "metabolic products" (*Stoffwechselproducte*), a platitudinous notion which has been called more sound than sense. Formerly they were termed secretory products, and I venture to say that it is better to remain with this name in order not to lose the analogy with glandular secretion.

There are thus two aspects to infection: the actual living parasites themselves, and their often poisonous secretions. In different diseases now one property, now the other, comes to the fore. In the case of the hematobiotic parasites formation of poisons is probably, as a rule, more important; in the case of those living in the organs the withdrawal of nutriment is more evident. The development of artificial nutritive media for bacteria has now provided us with a convenient tool for research and observation regarding all these questions.

It would be called carrying coals to Newcastle were I to sketch in London the beneficial effects which the application of these findings has exercised upon surgical practice. In the city where Lord Lister,[5] the man who by introducing antiseptic surgery brought about the greatest and most beneficial of all changes in medical science, still lives and works, everyone is aware how he anticipated the findings which the new theory of fermentative and septic processes confirmed. Before anyone had succeeded in demonstrating, with exact methods, the microbes active in various diseases, or in ascertaining their special mode of action, Lister, in a truly prophetic revelation, taught a method of protection against the action of putrefactive organisms. The opening of further regions of clinical medicine to the approach of the surgeon, and a revolution in the basis of therapeutics, have been the consequence. Lord Lister, whom I am proud to greet as an old friend, is now and always will be reckoned among the greatest benefactors of humanity. May he long remain at the head of the movement which he called into existence!

It remains for me to say a few words about the other great problem whose solution the whole world is awaiting with anxious impatience. I refer to the problem of immunity and its practical corollary, artificial immunization. It was another son of Albion who succeeded in introducing immunization as the definitive method of dealing with one of the most deadly of the infectious diseases. Jenner's great discovery has stood trial successfully, although not as completely as he had hoped. Vaccine is available to all, and vaccination, with governmental aid, is spreading continually. Pasteur worked in the same field, resolutely and boldly; he introduced the vaccines of fowl cholera, anthrax, and rabies. Others have followed him, and the new doctrine of antitoxins is continually acquiring more adherents. But it has not yet emerged from the conflict of opinions. Still less has the secret of immunity itself been revealed. Even if everything points to the view that immunity is based on the condition of cells and their contained fluids, and not on the serum or the humors—these being only a means of transport for the immunizing and infecting fluids—we must still be content with the hope that the next century will bring light and certainty on these points. The homeopathic notion that toxin and antitoxin are one and the same seems so foreign to our biological ideas that many experimental and practical proofs will be required before it can be admitted into the creed of the future. Before then we must succeed, by means of immunity, in finding a way of strengthening the cells in their fight with bacteria.

Let us, in conclusion, turn once more to the cells which build up the body, and which arise by proliferation within the body. These exhibit numerous analogies with microbes. They are also independent living beings, or, as Brücke said, elemental organisms implanted in the social structure of the body. They can be removed, transplanted, and grafted in new situations. If they increase in number and form a tumor, this can produce metastases by transplantation. But the process as such is always bound up with a certain number of living elements; it is always cellular in character. It is not the blood which makes a cell or a tumor; parent cells give rise to all new formations.

From this consideration I have for decades drawn the conclusion that the local action of cells, bound up with certain matricial parts, dominates pathological laws, and must also determine the practice of physicians and surgeons. Cellular pathology demands, above all, local treatment. It is with great pleasure that I see this conclusion continually becoming more widely accepted, with more or less conscious awareness of its nature. In surgery the consequence is the recommendation of early operation on, and destruction of, the focus of disease.

But cells also, just like bacteria, have chemical effects. Apart from the destruction due to absorption which they bring about, they also secrete chemical substances. These appear first as tissue fluids, passing later into the circulation. Thus arises a change in the composition of the fluids, and of the blood as well, in fact a dyscrasia. This is, as I have always attempted to make clear, a secondary dyscrasia, quite distinct from the primary dyscrasias whose localization was supposed by the humoral pathologists to give rise to local disease, in particular to tumors. According to my view, each dyscrasia is determined by the taking in of products of tissue secretion, whether they are called metabolic products or, according to the old dictum, recrementitious substances.

The tissue fluids, and the excreted material which is returned into the body, have of late years gained much importance. The sperm, which I myself have always indicated as the classical example of such a tissue juice and have made the prototype of secretion by cells of tumors and organs, has provided therapy with spermin, as the thyroid fluid provided thyroidin and thyroiodine. New substances, some resembling alkaloids, some albuminates, are isolated from various organs, experimentally tested, and technically applied. Thus injection therapy, or serum therapy, arose. We are not yet in a position to pass a final judgment on the results, although every unprejudiced observer must admit that they have in many cases been good. Experience will determine the value of these methods; we must learn to deduce the lasting theoretical truths from practice. That the source of all these substances and secretions is the cell activity of living tissue, and that its therapeutic or pathological action on the individual organs or tissues can thus accomplish nothing beyond exercising a regulatory influence on cell activity, must never be forgotten.

May the medical school of Charing Cross Hospital continue upon the new path with zeal and fortune! May its students also never forget that neither the physician nor the natural scientist can dispense with a cool head and a calm spirit, with practical observation and critical judgment.

Notes

For an account of the life and times of Rudolf Virchow, see Erwin H. Ackerknecht's *Rudolf Virchow: Doctor, Statesman, Anthropologist* (Madison, Wisc., 1953). In preparing the following biographical notes I have made use of the Haberling-Hübotter-Vierordt *Biographisches Lexikon der hervorragenden Ärzte aller Zeiten und Völker* (Berlin, 1929), the Delorme-Dechambre-Lereboullet *Dictionnaire encyclopédique des sciences médicales* (Paris, 1864–89), and the eleventh edition of the *Encyclopædia Britannica*.

Introduction

[1] *The Works of William Harvey, M.D., Translated from the Latin with a Life of the Author*, by Robert Willis, M.D. (London, 1847), p. 155.

[2] *Ibid.*, p. 156.

[3] W. H. S. Jones (*Philosophy and Medicine in Ancient Greece*, Bull. Hist. Med. Suppl. No. 8, 1946) says of hypotheses in Greek thought that the presence or absence of contradictions in the deductions drawn from hypotheses determined their validity, rather than an appeal to the phenomena. Modern science, writes Jones, begins with phenomena and ends with hypotheses, ancient philosophy began with hypotheses and ended nowhere; the chief difference between ancient and modern thought is that the former is deductive and the latter inductive. But was it not the Platonic school which stressed the necessity of "saving the phenomena"? Modern science is a highly hypothetical construction, and it is not true that a modern scientist begins with phenomena and ends with hypotheses; he begins and ends with a question involving a blend of both.

[4] *The Works of William Harvey*, p. 160.

[5] *Ibid.*, p. xli. See J. H. Woodger, *Biology and Language* (Cambridge, England, 1952).

[6] To suggest, as Woodger does, that Harvey regarded the heart and circulation like an intelligent plumber is to oversimplify matters considerably. In the letter to Riolan, Harvey states that the innate heat of the blood causes it to swell and rise "like bodies in a state of fermentation." The auricle, then being dilated, contracts and delivers its charge into the right ventricle. Systole ensuing, the charge is forced into the pulmonary artery, through the lungs, and into the left auricle, which, acting equally and synchronously

with the right, delivers the blood into the left ventricle, from whence blood is impelled into the arteries of the body. The "innate heat is the first cause of dilatation, and the primary dilatation is in the blood itself." The heart is not the source of the heat of the blood; rather it receives heat from the blood and hence is furnished with coronary arteries and veins. In addition there is a theological element in Harvey's outlook. Pagel ("Giordano Bruno: The Philosophy of Circles and the Circular Movement of the Blood," *J. Hist. Med. & Allied Sciences* 6: 116, 1951, and "Die Stellung Caesalpins und Harveys in der Entdeckung und Ideologie des Blutkreislaufes," *Sudhoffs Arch.* 37: 319, 1953) has shown that Harvey's work rested on two Aristotelian tenets, the perfection of circular motion and the parallelism between microcosm and macrocosm. The circulation of the blood was a reproduction on microcosmic lines of a pattern which characterized the universe as a whole. Harvey's work must be considered not only as an introduction of dynamic, quantitative ideas into static speculative anatomy but also as the crystallization of a scientifically formulated idea out of a mother liquor of philosophical-theological character.

[7] Woodger, *loc. cit.*

[8] The question here at issue is whether a hypothesis is *directly* verifiable or not. The sound of strange noises from a neighboring room might give rise to a number of hypotheses, the consequences of which could never settle a problem easily solved by opening the door and discovering, say, a bassoonist. There are many scientific hypotheses which have subsequently been directly verified. The discovery, for example, of certain small irregularities in the path of Uranus led to the hypothesis that these were due to the disturbing influence of an as yet unobserved planet. The hypothesis was well supported by precise calculations, but only when the new planet, Neptune, was itself observed could the hypothesis be said to have been *directly* verified. If Neptune had for some reason been inaccessible to observation, no amount of observation merely consistent with the hypothesis could have directly verified it. As a matter of fact, Leverrier made similar calculations to account for irregularities in the orbit of Mercury. These were likewise explainable by the hypothesis that there was an as yet unobserved planet in the neighborhood. It was tentatively named Vulcan. But no such planet has been found, and the explanation of the irregularities offered by relativity theory is considerably more elegant and powerful, since it accounts for other discrepancies in classical celestial dynamics.

[9] Claude Bernard, *Introduction a l'étude de la médecine expérimentale* (Paris, 1865). English translation by H. C. Greene (New York, 1949). In an address given at the Collège de France on the centenary of Bernard's birth, Bergson said: "Dans un cas comme dans l'autre nous nous trouvons devant un homme de génie qui a commencé par faire de grandes découvertes et qui s'est demandé ensuite comment il fallait s'y prendre pour les faire: marche paradoxale en apparence et pourtant seule naturelle, la manière in-

verse de procéder ayant été tentée beaucoup plus souvent et n'ayant jamais réussi. Deux fois seulement dans l'histoire de la science moderne, et pour les deux formes principales que notre connaissance de la nature a prises, l'esprit d'invention s'est replié sur lui-même pour s'analyser et pour déterminer ainsi les conditions générales de la découverte scientifique. Cet heureux mélange de spontanéité et de reflexion, de science et de philosophie, s'est produit les deux fois en France."

[10] He failed, of course, to convince all of his contemporaries. The French bacteriologist Maurice Arthus, for example, stated that a "fact" was absolute, categorical, and imperative, while a "theory" was a dogma based on articles of faith. Seek facts and classify them, he wrote, and you will be the workmen of science. Conceive or accept them and you will become its politicians. (In the Preface to his *De l'Anaphylaxie à l'immunité* (Paris, 1921), translated under the title "Philosophy of Scientific Investigation," H. Sigerist, *Bull. Hist. Med.* 14: 373, 1943.)

[11] Bernard, *Introduction* (Greene trans.), p. 23. This quotation and the following quotations are reprinted by permission of Abelard-Schuman Limited from Claude Bernard's *Experimental Medicine* (copyright 1927).

[12] *Ibid.*, p. 27.

[13] *Ibid.*, pp. 44 f.

[14] *Ibid.*, p. 152.

[15] Toward the middle of the nineteenth century a controversy between William Whewell and J. S. Mill highlighted this point. The three theses defended by Whewell were (1) the historical relativity of fact and theory, (2) the great importance of controversies about theory for the progress of scientific knowledge, and (3) the indispensable role of hypotheses in making scientific discoveries (E. W. Strong, "Whewell vs. J. S. Mill on Science," *J. Hist. Ideas*, April 1955). Not content with the "facts," which were so stressed by the empiricists of his day, Whewell enquired after the habits of thought and the implied ideas or assumptions standing behind the facts. According to Whewell, hypotheses and theories introduced new *principles of order* into the facts of observation. Mill, on the other hand, insisted that these new principles of order were simply generalizations based on particular facts. Whewell's emphasis on the creative element in scientific procedure, and his insistence that facts were always *interpreted* facts, placed him in opposition to the prevailing trend of British empiricism, and it is probably for this reason that he has not received the recognition that has been given to Mill. Whewell called this procedure "discoverer's logic" and used the term induction for want of a better. It has also been called "hypothetical deduction," "abduction" (Peirce), "diagnosis" (Ducasse), and "creative induction" (L. de Broglie, "Déduction et induction dans la recherche scientifique," *Scientia* 90: 1, 1955). Lukasiewicz calls it "reduction," in order to make the distinction from ordinary induction and deduction clear. In a discussion of "reduction" Bochenski (*Die Zeitgenössischen Denkmethoden,*

Bern, 1954) makes it plain that this procedure enables a scientist not only to pass from observation generalizations to hypothetical statements of higher order, but also to move freely at the level of observation like a historian, an archeologist, or even, one might add, a detective.

[16] It is easy to become confused as to level and direction when moving among these statements, and to invert their order of priority. In his system of general semantics Korzybski not only inverted the order but introduced a logical circle which made the highest order of abstraction (i.e. the hypothetical structures of physical science) at the same time the foundation of the lower orders (since the "mad dance" of electrons was supposed to be the fundamental basis from which the nervous system constructed its "abstractions"). Cf. Max Black, *Language and Philosophy* (Ithaca, N.Y., 1949).

[17] *Rudolf Virchow: Briefe an seine Eltern,* edited by Marie Rabl (Leipzig, 1907), letter dated August 27, 1845.

[18] "Die Universalität von Rudolf Virchows Lebenswerk," *Virchows Archiv* 322: 221, 1952.

[19] "The Speculative Basis of Modern Pathology," *Bull. Hist. Med.* 18: 1, 1945.

[20] Rudolf Virchow als Systematiker und Philosoph," *Virchows Archiv* 300: 517, 1937.

[21] *Virchows Cellularpathologie,* Protoplasma Monographien (Berlin, 1938).

[22] Virchow, "Specifiker und Specifisches," *Virchows Archiv* 6: 1, 1854.

[23] *Ibid.*

[24] For current attacks on the second hypothesis see Ovlitt's review of O. B. Lepeshinskaya's book *The Origin of Protoplasmic Cells and the Role of the Protoplasm in the Organism,* in the *American Review of Soviet Medicine,* 4: 472, 1947, and the discussion between Busse-Grawitz and Rössle in the *Zentralbl. f. allg. Path. u. path. Anat.* 96: 376, 1957.

[25] "Über die Standpunkte in der wissenschaftlichen Medicin," *Virchows Archiv* 1: 3, 1847.

[26] "Die naturwissenschaftliche Methode und die Standpunkte in der Therapie," *Virchows Archiv* 2: 3, 1849.

[27] *Hundert Jahre allgemeiner Pathologie* (Berlin, 1895).

[28] "Die naturwissenschaftliche Methode" (1849).

[29] "Über die Standpunkte" (1847).

[30] Virchow, *Die Einheitsbestrebungen in der wissenschaftlichen Medicin* (Berlin, G. Reimer), 1849.

[31] *Medical Observations Concerning the History and the Cure of Acute Diseases,* translated from Latin by R. G. Latham (London, 1848) Vol. I, Preface to the third edition.

[32] "Die naturwissenschaftliche Methode" (1849).

[33] *Hundert Jahre allgemeiner Pathologie* (1895).

[34] *Die Einheitsbestrebungen* (1849).

[35] "Die naturwissenschaftliche Methode" (1849).

[36] *Über die mechanische Auffassung des Lebens,* in *Vier Reden über Leben und Kranksein; unveränderter Abdruck* (Berlin, 1862).

[37] "Cellularpathologie," *Virchows Archiv* 8: 1, 1855.

[38] *Hundert Jahre allgemeiner Pathologie* (1895).

[39] *Die Gründung der Berliner Universität und der Übergang aus dem philosophischen in das naturwissenschaftliche Zeitalter* (Berlin, 1893).

[40] *Die Einheitsbestrebungen* (1849).

[41] "Die naturwissenschaftliche Methode" (1849).

Standpoints in Scientific Medicine

[1] Jean Cruveilhier (1791–1874), the son of a military physician in the army of the Republic, was born in Limoges. At the insistence of his father he reluctantly entered into the study of medicine and attained his doctorate in Paris at the age of twenty-five. He became professor of surgery at Montpellier soon after, through the persistence of his father and the good offices of Dupuytren. In 1825 he was called to Paris as professor of descriptive anatomy, and in 1836 became professor of pathological anatomy, remaining in this post for thirty years.

[2] Victor Alexander Bochdalek (1801–83) was professor of anatomy at the University of Prague. Very little is known of his life.

[3] Carl Freiherr von Rokitansky (1804–74) was born at Königgrätz in Bohemia and studied medicine in Prague and Vienna. He became professor at the general hospital in Vienna in 1844, and his *Handbuch der pathologische Anatomie* was published in 1842–46. It was based on an enormous amount of observational data, but his explanations of pathological events rested on humoralistic views. He renounced these shortly after Virchow's criticism of his book appeared. Besides being an acute and tireless observer, Rokitansky had a talent for philosophical analysis and speculation which Lange comments on in his *History of Materialism.*

Scientific Method and Therapeutic Standpoints

[1] William Harvey (1578–1657) was born in Kent, was educated at Cambridge University, and received a doctorate in medicine from the University of Padua in 1602. His investigations on the heart and circulation were published in Frankfurt a.M. in 1628. Twenty-three years later his studies on the generation of animals established the theory of the origin of all living things from eggs. Virchow's "omnis cellula a cellula" derives from Harvey's "omne vivum ex ovo."

Albrecht von Haller (1708–77) was born in Bern of a prominent family.

An eager sickly precocious child, he began to study medicine at the University of Tübingen in his fifteenth year. He received his doctorate from the University of Leyden, and later studied in London and Paris. Returning to his native city he tried unsuccessfully to obtain a professorship of history and a position in the city hospital, but was regarded as too much the scholar for the latter and too much the practical man for the former. He obtained a post at the library and soon became known as a poet, botanist, and anatomist. He was called to the newly founded University of Göttingen as professor of anatomy, surgery, and botany, and at the age of twenty-eight became head of the entire University. During his stay he carried out numerous experiments on the effect of mechanical, thermal, electrical, and chemical stimuli on the tissues. He held that the nerves possessed "sensibility" and the muscles "irritability," and is regarded as one of the founders of experimental physiology.

Sir Charles Bell (1774–1842), brother of the surgeon John Bell, was born in Edinburgh, Scotland, and studied medicine in Edinburgh. While still students he and his brother became known for their published work on anatomy. In 1809, and again in greater detail in 1821, he described the functions of the anterior and posterior nerve roots.

François Magendie (1783–1855) was born in Bordeaux and studied medicine in Paris. In 1836 he became professor of physiology and general pathology at the Collège de France. He regarded experimentation as the chief source of knowledge, and founded a journal of experimental physiology (Paris, 1821–31). He shares with Bell credit for discovering the function of the nerve roots.

Johannes Müller (1801–58) was born in Coblenz. The son of a shoemaker, he became one of the greatest biologists of all time. He studied medicine at Bonn and won a prize, as a student, with his work on fetal respiration. In 1833 he became professor of anatomy and physiology in Berlin. His work covers a very wide range embracing human and comparative anatomy, experimental physiology, developmental anatomy, pathological anatomy, and physiological chemistry. He developed the doctrine of reflexes, studied the mechanism of voice production, promoted the use of the microscope in anatomical investigations, and wrote on the structure of tumors. Schwann, Virchow, du Bois-Reymond, and von Helmholtz were only a few of his students who became famous.

[2] Johann Nepomuk von Ringseis (1785–1880) was an opponent of Virchow who regarded disease as a consequence of original sin. Jacob Joseph Görres (1776–1848) was a pietist and nature-philosopher.

[3] Josef Skoda (1805–81) was professor of medicine at Vienna.

[4] Matheo-Jose-Bonaventure Orfila (1787–1853) was professor of legal medicine, and later of chemistry, at Paris. He was best known for his work in toxicology.

[5] Samuel Hahnemann (1755–1843), the founder of homeopathy, was born in Saxony and educated in medicine at Leipzig, Vienna, and Erlangen.

[6] Justus Freiherr von Liebig (1803–73) was professor of chemistry, and founder of the first great chemical laboratory, at Giessen. He was later a professor at Munich.

[7] Carl (1805–71) and Eilhard (1794–1863) Mitscherlich were professors of pharmacology and chemistry, respectively, at Berlin.

[8] Johann Gottfried Rademacher (1772–1850) was born in Westphalia and studied medicine in Jena and Berlin. He was the founder of "Erfahrungsheillehre," a variant of the Paracelsian doctrine of signatures. He held that the outward manifestations of disease gave no true knowledge of their real nature. This knowledge could be obtained only by a study of therapeutic agents, and diseases could be understood and classified only in terms of the agents most effective against them.

[9] François Joseph Victor Broussais (1772–1838), born in St.-Malo, received his first instruction in medicine from his father and his medical degree at Paris. He became professor of general pathology at the Academy of Medicine in Paris in 1831.

[10] Gesellschaft für wissenschaftliche Medicin zu Berlin, Sitzung vom 28 July, 1847.

[11] Salomon Neumann (1819–1908) was born in Pyritz (Pomerania), studied in Berlin and Halle, and became widely known for his work in public health and preventive medicine. The book to which Virchow refers, *Die öffentliche Gesundheitspflege und das Eigenthum*, was published in Berlin in 1847.

Cellular Pathology

[1] Here, as elsewhere, when Virchow refers to the Archives he means the *Archiv für pathologische Anatomie und Physiologie und für klinische Medizin*, known since his death as *Virchows Archiv*.

[2] Alfred-Armand-Louis-Marie Velpeau (1795–1867), son of a poor handworker, was born in Brèche, France. He studied medicine in Tours, then in Paris, where he became a prominent surgeon. He was a prodigious worker and his publications cover a wide range of topics in general surgery and pathology. The sentence he is said to have muttered on his deathbed— "Il ne faut pas être paresseux; travaillons toujours!"—recalls the title of Virchow's Gymnasium composition: "Ein Leben voller Mühe ist keine Last sondern eine Wohltat."

[3] Franz Schuh, born in Vienna in 1804, was a surgeon well known for his biting and witty style. He was greatly interested in autopsy and surgical pathology. The first book, referred to by Virchow, *Über die Erkenntnis der Pseudoplasmen*, was published in Vienna in 1851, and reviewed by Virchow

in the *Jahresberichte über die Fortschritte der gesamten Medicin*, 4:194, 1851. The second book, *Pathologie und Therapie der Pseudoplasmen*, appeared in 1854. Abnormal growths of many kinds, including those now classified as neoplasms and granulomas, were designated "Pseudoplasmen."

[4] "And Homer's sun, behold, it smiles on us as well."

[5] Pierre Paul Broca (1824–80), was an anatomist and professor of surgical pathology at Paris. His "Mémoire sur l'anatomie pathologique du cancer," which won the Portal prize, appears in the *Mém. de l'Acad. de Méd.*, XVI (1852), 453. Broca was also the founder of the Anthropological Society of Paris.

[6] John Hughes Bennett (1812–75) was born in London and studied medicine at Edinburgh, Paris, and several German universities. He became professor of medicine at the University of Edinburgh. His book *Cancerous and Other Growths*, to which Virchow refers, appeared in 1849.

[7] "Spezifisches und Spezifiker," *Virchows Archiv*, 6:9, 1854.

[8] Georges Leopold Cuvier (1769–1832), zoologist, anatomist, paleontologist, and geologist, was born in Montbéliard, France, and studied at Stuttgart under Schiller. His book *Discours sur les révolutions de la surface du globe*, to which Virchow refers, was published in 1828.

[9] Cf. Virchow's *Handbuch der speciellen Pathologie und Therapie*.

[10] Josef Engel (1816–99) was born in Vienna, where he studied and received his doctorate. He was successively professor of pathological anatomy in Prague and professor at the Medizinisch-chirurgische Josefs-Akademie in Vienna. His book *Specielle pathologische Anatomie* was published in Vienna in 1856.

[11] Richard Ladislaus Heschl (1824–81), born in Wellsdorf, Steiermark, studied medicine in Vienna and became Rokitansky's assistant. He was professor of pathological anatomy first in Krakau, then in Graz.

[12] Hermann Lebert (1813–78), born in Breslau, studied medicine and botany in Berlin and Zurich, practiced and taught in Paris. He was one of the first to put the microscope to good use in pathology.

[13] Friedrich Günsburg (1820–59) was born in Breslau. He wrote a number of important papers on pathology, in addition to founding the *Zeitschrift für klinische Medizin*, before his untimely death. Virchow refers to his book *Das Epithelialgewebe des menschlichen Körpers*, published in Bonn in 1854.

[14] "Ernährungseinheiten und Krankheitsherde," *Virchows Archiv*, 4: 375, 1852.

[15] Presumably Bernard Seyfert (1817–70), the obstetrician.

[16] *Handbuch der speciellen Pathologie und Therapie*.

[17] Gustav-Adolph Spiess (1802–75) was born in Duisburg and received his doctorate at Heidelberg. He practiced medicine in Frankfurt a.M. and gained renown in the philosophy of science, general pathology, and public

health. His book *Zur Lehre von der Entzündung*, to which Virchow refers, was published in 1854.

[18] Johann Christian Reil (1759–1813), born in East Friesland, studied at Göttingen and Halle. In 1810 he was called to Berlin as professor of clinical medicine. His famous essay on vitalism, *Von der Lebenskraft*, was published in the first volume (1796) of the *Archiv für die Physiologie*, which he founded and edited for nineteen years. In addition to anatomy and physiology he was interested in psychiatry and attempted, unsuccessfully, to found psychiatric institutes in Halle and Berlin.

[19] Carl Heinrich Schultz (1798–1871) changed his name to Schultz-Schultzenstein to avoid being confused with his colleague in botany C. H. Schultz. Born in Alt-Ruppin, he received his doctorate in Berlin. He held to a transcendental standpoint in physiology and pathology and was, in consequence, involved in many controversies with Virchow, du Bois-Reymond, Müller, and others.

[20] *Handbuch der speciellen Pathologie und Therapie*, I, 272.

[21] Konrad Eckhard (1822–1905) was born in Hamburg and studied in Marburg, Berlin, and Giessen. His book *Grundzüge der Physiologie des Nervensystems*, to which Virchow refers, was published in Giessen in 1854.

[22] Franz von Leydig (1821–1908), born in Rothenburg, studied philosophy in Munich and medicine in Würzburg. He became professor of zoology and comparative anatomy at Tübingen, and later at Bonn, and was known for his work on the development and structure of lower animals.

[23] Probably Rudolph Wagner (1805–64), the anatomist and physiologist.

[24] Guillaume-Benjamin-Amand Duchenne (1806–75), born in Boulogne, studied in Paris. A clinical neurologist and a neurophysiologist, he made extensive and original investigations of the effect of electrical stimuli on the tissues.

[25] Karl Gotthelf Lehmann (1812–63) was professor of physiological chemistry at Leipzig, and later professor of chemistry at Jena.

[26] Über parenchymatöse Entzündung," *Virchows Archiv*, 4:261, 1852.

[27] *Ibid.*

[28] Moritz Heinrich Romberg (1795–1873), born in Meiningen, studied in Berlin, where he became professor of special pathology and therapy in 1845. He was a neural pathologist, a representative of the school whose doctrines Virchow was attacking.

[29] Friedrich Gustav Henle (1809–85), born in Fürth, studied at Bonn under Johannes Müller, and at Berlin. He was imprisoned in 1835 because of his political activities, but pardoned thanks to the intervention of Alexander von Humboldt. A zoologist, anatomist, and pathologist, he founded the *Zeitschrift für rationelle Medicin*.

[30] See note 1, p. 252.

[31] Ludwig Traube (1818–76), born in Ratibor, studied medicine in Berlin. A clinician and neurologist, he founded, together with Virchow and Reinhardt, the journal *Beiträge zur experimentellen Pathologie.*

[32] Albrecht von Graefe (1828–70), born in Berlin, was a brilliant student who entered the University to study medicine at the age of sixteen. He became professor of ophthalmology at the University of Berlin, and founder of the *Archiv für Ophthalmologie.*

[33] Moritz Schiff (1823–96), born in Frankfurt a.M., studied in Heidelberg, Berlin, and Göttingen. He became professor of physiology in Florence and Geneva, and was known for his work in ornithology and neurology.

[34] See note 1, pp. 251–52.

[35] Verein für gemeinschaftliche Arbeiten zur Förderung der wissenschaftlichen Heilkunde.

Atoms and Individuals

[1] "Where now, as our wise ones say, a soulless ball of fire rotates, Helios in quiet majesty once guided his golden chariot. Oreads filled these heights, a Dryad lived in every tree, from the urns of lovely Naiads sprang the silvery foam of streams. Ah! from that warm and living picture only the shadow remains. Like the dead stroke of the pendulum, bereft of gods, Nature meanly serves the rule of gravity." Schiller, "Die Götter Griechenlands."

[2] "Therefore care has been taken that trees do not grow to the heavens."

[3] Matthias Jakob Schleiden (1804–81), born in Hamburg, first studied jurisprudence in Heidelberg, but after a few years of practice began the study of natural science in Göttingen and later continued his studies in Berlin. He became professor and director of the botanical garden in Jena in 1839. He taught botany, plant chemistry, and anthropology in Dresden and Dorpat. His investigations of plant cells were first published in 1837–38.

[4] Theodor Schwann (1810–82), born in Neuss, studied at Bonn, Würzburg, and Berlin, pursuing mathematics and philosophy as well as medicine. Others had described cells before him, but he emphasized their similarity in plants and animals, as well as the derivation of animal tissues from cells, carrying out investigations on young embryos to demonstrate this point. He was also the discoverer of gastric pepsin. His book *Mikroscopische Untersuchungen über die Übereinstimmungen der Structur und dem Wachstum der Tiere und Pflanzen* was published in Berlin in 1839.

[5] Abraham Trembley (1700–1784) was a Swiss naturalist. His *Mémoires pour servir à l'histoire d'un genre de polypes d'eau douce* was published in Leyden in 1744.

[6] Karl Vogt (1817–95), born in Giessen, studied in Bern, Paris, and Giessen. He was forced to flee Germany because of his parliamentary activi-

ties, and while in exile published a zoological satire, *Untersuchung über Thierstaaten* (Frankfurt, 1851). Vogt was an explorer, a geologist, a zoologist, and a proponent of materialism and Darwinism. His book *Ocean und Mittelmeer*, to which Virchow refers, was published in 1848.

Standpoints in Scientific Medicine [1877]

[1] Benno Reinhardt (1819–52) was born in Mecklenburg, studied in Berlin and Halle, and followed Virchow as prosector at the Charité in Berlin. He was co-founder of the *Archiv für pathologische Anatomie, Physiologie und für klinische Medizin*.

[2] "Ernährungseinheiten und Krankheitsherde," *Virchows Archiv* 4:375, 1852.

The Place of Pathology among the Biological Sciences

[1] The Royal Society.

[2] Georg Ernst Stahl (1660–1734) studied medicine in Jena. Called to Halle as professor of medicine in 1694, he taught, in opposition to the iatrochemical and iatrophysical doctrines then current, his system of Animism. Stahl's "anima" is related to the "physis" of Hippocrates. He reacted against the doctrines of those who, basing themselves on the new Cartesian philosophy, wanted to explain life in terms of mechanics or chemistry. According to Stahl it was the "anima" which produced disease by disturbing vital processes. In support of his position, he pointed out the effect of the emotions on bodily processes.

[3] John Hunter (1728–93), born in Lanarkshire, had little formal education and learned anatomy and medicine largely through studying under his brother William and Sir Percival Pott. He became an accomplished surgeon, anatomist, physiologist, and zoologist. A brilliant experimenter, he once wrote to Edward Jenner, "I think your solution is just; but why think? why not try the experiment?" Hunter taught that life was a principle independent of structure and, like Harvey, considered the blood to possess a vitality of its own.

[4] Francis Glisson (1597–1677), born in Rampisham, studied medicine at Cambridge, where he became professor of medicine. He regarded "irritability," i.e. the capability of being affected by stimuli, as a basic characteristic of all substances. His book *De Rachitete Sive Morbo Puerili, Qui Vulgo the Rickets Dicitur*, to which Virchow refers, was published in 1660, the *Anatomia Hepatis* in 1654.

[5] *Virchows Archiv* 14:1, 1858.

[6] *Virchows Archiv* 5:410, 1853.

[7] "Treatise on the nature of energized substance, or, on natural life and its three chief faculties, perceptive, appetitive, and motive."

⁸ *Biarchia* is from *biarches*, meaning "supplying what is necessary for life." *Biusia* means "the substance of life"; *vita substantialis vel vitae substantia* means "substantial life or the substance of life." *Archaeus* is the latinized form of the Greek *archaios*, meaning "principle" (of life). *Vis plastica* means "plastic force."

⁹ Thomas Willis (1621–75), born in Wiltshire, studied at Oxford, where he took the degree of bachelor of medicine in 1646 and became professor of natural philosophy in 1660. He was admired for his work in anatomy, chemistry, and experimental philosophy, as well as for the elegance and purity of his Latin style. He began the practice of medicine in 1666.

¹⁰ Hermann Boerhaave (1668–1738) was born near Leyden, where he took his degree in philosophy in 1689 with a dissertation on the distinction between the body and the mind in which he attacked Epicurus, Hobbes, and Spinoza. Four years later he received his degree in medicine at Harderwyck in Guelderland. He became professor of medicine and botany at Leyden and inaugurated the modern system of clinical instruction; later he took over the chair of chemistry as well. Among others, Peter the Great studied under him.

¹¹ Hieronymus Davides Gaubius (1705–80), born in Heidelberg, studied medicine at Harderwyck and Leyden. First a lecturer in chemistry at Leyden, he became professor of medicine in 1734, presenting an inaugural lecture entitled "Oratio de Vana Vitae Longae a Chemicis Promissa Exspectatione." His *Institutiones Pathologiae Medicinalis* was published in 1758.

¹² *Actio propria sic dicta* means "so-called special action"; *motus activus*, "active motion"; *principium dividendi*, "principle of division."

¹³ "That which lives through itself lives a life dependent on no other creature but itself. For this is what the words 'vivere per se' mean."

¹⁴ William Hewson (1739–74), born in Northumberland, studied in London, Paris, and Edinburgh. He was prosector under the brothers Hunter.

¹⁵ See note 19, p. 255.

¹⁶ "Crasis," a mixing.

¹⁷ Marie Jean Pierre Flourens (1794–1867) received his doctorate at Montpellier. A physiologist and neurologist, he became a member of the Academy and a peer of France.

¹⁸ John Brown (1735–78), born in Berwickshire, Scotland, studied divinity and medicine at Edinburgh. In the Brownian or Brunonian System health consisted in an equilibrium between irritability and stimulation; therapy, accordingly, involved increasing or decreasing the degree of stimulation.

¹⁹ Johann Lucas Schönlein (1793–1864) was professor of special pathology and therapy at Freiburg i. Br.

²⁰ Emil du Bois-Reymond (1818–96), born in Berlin, studied medicine

under Johannes Müller at the University and succeeded Müller as professor of physiology. He wrote on philosophical problems as well as on comparative anatomy and physiology.

[21] Giovanni Battista Morgagni (1682–1771), born at Forli, studied medicine and philosophy at Bologna, and held the chair of medicine at Padua from 1712 to 1771. In 1761 he brought out his *De Sedibus et Causis Morborum per Anatomen Indigatis*, which directed medicine toward clinical-pathological correlation.

[22] Marie François Xavier Bichat (1771–1802), born at Thoirette, studied in Lyons and Paris.

One Hundred Years of General Pathology

[1] Kos and Knidos were rival medical schools of ancient Greece. The Hippocratic doctrines are associated with Kos.

[2] Claudius Galenus, the most influential of the ancient medical writers, was active in Rome in the second century A.D. He wrote a large number of original treatises and commentaries on logic, science, and medicine.

[3] Andreas Vesalius (1514–64), a native of Brussels, taught at Padua, Bologna, and Pisa. He was the author of a comprehensive, systematic treatise which corrected many of the errors of Galenic anatomy. This he had accomplished at the age of twenty-eight; for the rest of his life he was in the service of the Spanish imperial house.

[4] Theophrast Bombast von Hohenheim, self-styled Paracelsus (1490–1591), was born in the canton Schwyz, studied at Basel and Würzburg, worked in the Tirolean mines of the Fuggers, and came to believe that positive knowledge of nature must be obtained at first hand. To read the book of nature, he said, the physician must walk over the leaves. Later he taught and practiced in Basel, where he met with so much resistance that he had to leave in haste. For the next twelve years he wandered over Germany, finally settling down in Salzburg under the protection of the archbishop. His death was attributed by his enemies to a drunken debauch; others said that he was thrown from a steep place by agents of the physicians or apothecaries, both of whom he had harassed. Medicine, for Paracelsus, was based on the general relationship of man to nature as a whole.

[5] Marcello Malpighi (1628–94) was born near Bologna, where he studied medicine and was granted his doctorate in 1653. He was one of the first to apply the microscope to the study of living structures, and in 1661 (four years after Harvey's death) described the capillary circulation *in vivo*.

[6] Antony van Leeuwenhoek (1632–1723), a Dutch microscopist born at Delft, confirmed Malpighi's discovery of the capillary circulation, and gave the first accurate description of red blood cells in men, frogs, and fishes.

[7] Of the medical school at Montpellier it was said, *olim Cous nunc Monspelliensis Hippocrates*. In 1295 Arnold of Villanova taught the Hippocratic tradition there; in the seventeenth century the school combated the iatromechanists; and in the eighteenth century Théophile Bordeu (1722–76), Joseph Barthez (1734–78) and Charles L. Dumas (1765–1813) supported the vitalistic positions.

[8] Anthelme-Balthasar Richerand (1779–1840), surgeon, writer, and philosopher, edited the works of Bordeu in 1818.

[9] Luigi Galvani (1737–98) was born at Bologna and educated at the university, where he was appointed public lecturer in anatomy in 1762. His theory of animal electricity is enunciated in a treatise *De Viribus Electricitatis in Motu Musculari Commentarius*, published in 1791. He lost his professorship in 1797, when he refused to take an oath of allegiance to the Cisalpine Republic, and died before he could be reinstated.

[10] Friedrich (or Franz) Anton Mesmer (1733–1815) studied medicine in Vienna, but became interested in astrology and supposed that the force exerted by the stars on men might be of electrical or magnetic character. His first treatments involved stroking the body with magnets. In Paris he attracted crowds of patients, and in the dimly lit consulting rooms they sat around a vat of chemical ingredients while Mesmer, clad as a magician, glided about making passes with his hands or stroking and eyeing the sufferers. A governmental commission, including Benjamin Franklin, admitted the phenomena produced but contested Mesmer's theory of animal magnetism.

[11] Andreas Röschlaub (1787–1835) studied medicine in Bamberg and Würzburg, and served as professor of pathology and clinical medicine at Bamberg, then at Munich. He translated Brown's works into German.

[12] Matthew Baillie (1761–1823), born in Scotland, was a nephew of John and William Hunter. After William Hunter's death Baillie inherited his house, his anatomical theater and museum, and an annual income of one hundred pounds. In 1793 he published the atlas *The Morbid Human Anatomy of Some of the Most Important Parts of the Human Body*, to which Virchow refers.

[13] Johann Nathanael Lieberkühn (1711–56) was first a student of theology, then studied medicine under Boerhaave and Gaubius at Leyden. His *De Fabrica et Actione Villorum et Intestorum Tenuium* was published in 1745.

[14] Johann Gottlieb Walter (1734–1818) was professor of anatomy at Frankfurt a.O. and professor of obstetrics at the Charité.

[15] Johann Friedrich Meckel, the elder (1724–74), was professor of anatomy, botany, and obstetrics at Berlin. His *Physiologische und anatomische Abhandlungen von ungewöhnlicher Erweiterung des Herzens und der Spannadern des Angesichts*, to which Virchow refers, was published in 1755.

[16] Caspar Friedrich Wolff (1733–94) was professor of anatomy and physiology at the academy of St. Petersburg.

[17] Christoph Wilhelm Hufeland (1762–1836).

[18] Virchow refers here to von Humboldt's essay "Die Lebenskraft, oder der rhodische Genius," a philosophical allegory contributed in June 1795 to Schiller's new periodical *Die Hören.* Döllinger, von Walther, Schönlein, and Johannes Müller were temporarily attracted by the work of the naturephilosophers.

[19] Karl Asmund Rudolphi (1771–1832) was director of the anatomical institute at Berlin.

[20] Johann Friedrich Meckel, the younger (1781–1833).

[21] René Théophile Laennec (1781–1826). His *De l'Auscultation médiate ou traité du diagnostic des maladies des poumons et du cœur, fondé principalement sur ce nouveau moyen d'exploration* was published in 1819.

[22] Guillaume Dupuytren (1778–1835).

[23] Leopold Auenbrugger (1722–1809) was chief physician at the Spanish Hospital in Vienna, where his *Inventum Novum ex Percussione Thoracic Humani, ut Signo, Abstrusos Interni Pectoris Morbos Detegendi* was published in 1761.

[24] Gabriel Andral (1797–1876) was professor of general pathology and therapy at Paris. His *Traité d'anatomie pathologique* was published in 1829, and his *Essai d'hématologie pathologique* in 1843.

[25] Louis Denis Gavarret (1809–90) was professor of medical physics at Paris.

[26] See note 9, p. 253.

[27] Marshall Hall (1790–1857), born in Nottingham, studied medicine chiefly in Edinburgh, although he visited medical centers in Paris, Berlin, and Göttingen. His paper "On the Reflex Function of the Medulla Oblongata and Medulla Spinalis" appeared in 1832.

[28] Johann Friedrich Blumenbach (1752–1840), born in Gotha, studied medicine at Jena and Göttingen, and became professor of medicine at the latter university in 1778. He was a physiologist, a comparative anatomist, and an anthropologist whose division of the human race into five families— the Caucasian, the Mongolian, the Malayan, the Negro, and the American— is still generally accepted.

[29] Lorenz Oken (1779–1851) was professor of physiology at Munich, and professor of zoology at Erlangen.

[30] Ignatius Döllinger (1770–1841) was professor of anatomy and physiology at Würzburg, and later at Munich.

[31] Carl Ernst von Baer (1792–1876) taught at St. Petersburg for more than thirty years. Anatomist, physiologist, zoologist, and anthropologist, he is best known for his work on the mammalian ovum.

[32] Carl Wilhelm Stark (1787–1845) was professor of medicine at Jena

and author of *Allgemeine Pathologie oder Allgemeine Naturlehre der Krankheit* (Leipzig, 1838, 1844).

[33] Karl Friedrich Heusinger (1792–1883) later became professor of medicine at Marburg.

[34] Johann Wagner (1800–1833).

[35] Alois Rudolf Vetter (1765–1806) was famous for his *Aphorismen aus der pathologischen Anatomie* (Vienna, 1803).

[36] Franz Unger (1800–1870) was professor of plant physiology in Vienna and author of *Die Exantheme der Pflanzen* (Vienna, 1833).

[37] Agostino Bassi (1773–1856).

[38] Robert Remak (1815–65), histologist, embryologist, and neurologist.

[39] Ferdinand Jahn (1804–59) was directing physician at the George hospital in Meiningen.

[40] Carl Reinhold Wunderlich (1815–77) was professor of medicine at Leipzig. Virchow refers to the founding of the *Archiv für physiologische Heilkunde* in 1842.

[41] Rudolf Hermann Lotze (1817–81) studied philosophy and natural sciences at Leipzig, although officially a student of medicine. He became professor of philosophy at Göttingen and published a series of books aimed at the study of physical and mental phenomena of the human organism, in health and disease, according to principles used in the investigation of inorganic phenomena.

[42] Justus Friedrich Carl Hecker (1795–1850), professor of the history of medicine at Berlin, was a student of the history of the interaction of disease and society.

[43] Gerhard van Swieten (1700–1772).

[44] Anton de Haen (1704–76).

[45] Maximilian Stoll (1742–88).

[46] Burkhard Eble (1799–1839).

[47] Philipp Phoebus (1804–80). His most important work was done in botany and pharmacy.

[48] Robert Froriep (1828–61).

[49] Christian Gottfried Ehrenberg (1795–1876) was professor of medicine at Berlin.

[50] Gabriel Gustav Valentin (1810–83) was professor of physiology at Bern.

[51] Karl Bogislaus Reichert (1811–83).

[52] Heinrich Wilhelm Waldeyer (1836–1921).

[53] Rudolf Albert von Kölliker (1817–1905) was professor of anatomy, microscopy, and embryology at Würzburg.

[54] Carl Theodor von Siebold (1804–85) was professor of physiology, comparative anatomy, human anatomy, and zoology at Munich.

[55] Karl Georg Friedrich Leuckart (1823–98) was professor of zoology and comparative anatomy at Giessen and Leipzig. His *Untersuchungen über Trichina Spiralis* appeared in 1861.

[56] Karl Heitzmann (1836–96) studied in Budapest and Vienna, and practiced in New York. He combated the cell doctrine in a lecture in 1883 at the Berlin Medical Society, and also in an article "The Cell Doctrine in the Light of Recent Investigations," *New York Medical Journal*, 1877.

[57] Paul Grawitz (1850–1932).

[58] Karl von Pfeufer (1806–69) was later professor of medicine at Zurich.

[59] Ludwig Güterbock (1817–95).

[60] Gottlieb Gluge (1812–98) was later professor at Brussels. Virchow refers to his doctor's thesis, published in Berlin in 1835.

[61] Friedrich von Recklinghausen (1833–1910) was later professor of pathological anatomy at Würzburg, and after 1872 at Strassburg.

[62] Julius Cohnheim (1839–84) was professor of pathological anatomy at Kiel, Breslau, and Leipzig.

[63] Ferdinand Julius Cohn (1828–98) was professor of botany at Breslau.

[64] "Krankheitswesen und Krankheitsursachen," *Virchows Archiv* 79:1, 1880.

[65] Ludwig Brieger (1849–1919). His *Über Ptomaine* was published in 1885–86.

[66] Francesco Selmi (1817–81), professor of pharmaceutical chemistry at Bologna.

[67] Emil von Behring (1854–1917).

Recent Progress in Science

[1] "Morgagni and the Anatomic Concept," by Rudolf Virchow. Translated by R. E. Schlueter and John Auer. *Bull. Hist. Med.* 7: 975, 1939.

[2] *Bastian Festschrift* (Berlin, 1896).

[3] Wilhelm Roux (1850–1924) was director of the first institute for developmental mechanics in Germany, at Giessen.

[4] Gerhard Armauer Hansen (1841–1912) of Bergen, Norway. His "Studien über den Bacillus Leprae" appeared in *Virchows Archiv* in 1882.

[5] Joseph Lister (1827–1912). The first of his publications on antiseptic surgery, "On a New Method of Treating Compound Fracture, Abscess etc. with Observations in the Conditions of Suppuration," appeared in 1867.

German Titles and Sources of Articles Translated

"Über die Standpunkte in der wissenschaftlichen Medicin," *Virchows Archiv* 1:3, 1847

"Wissenschaftliche Methode und therapeutische Standpunkte," *Virchows Archiv* 2:3, 1849

Der Mensch. Einheitsbestrebungen in der wissenschaftlichen Medicin (Berlin, 1849)

"Cellular-Pathologie," *Virchows Archiv* 8:1, 1855

"Über die mechanische Auffassung des Lebens," in *Vier Reden über Leben und Kranksein* (Berlin, 1862)

"Atome und Individuen," in the same

"Über die Standpunkte in der wissenschaftlichen Medicin," *Virchows Archiv* 70:1, 1877

"Die Stellung der Pathologie unter den biologischen Wissenschaften," *Berliner klinische Wochenschrift* 30:321, 1893

Hundert Jahre allgemeiner Pathologie (Berlin, 1895)

"Die neueren Fortschritte in der Wissenschaft und ihr Einfluss auf Medicin und Chirurgie," *Berliner klinische Wochenschrift* 35:897, 1898

Index

DATE

HETERICK MEMORIAL LIBRARY
610 V81dEr   onuu
Virchow, Rudolf Lud/Disease, life, and m

3 5111 00148 7838